G000320200

INTELLIGENT EXERCISE
WITH
PILATES & YOGA

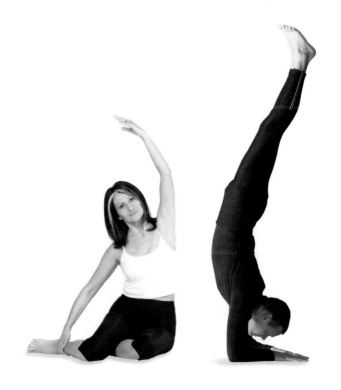

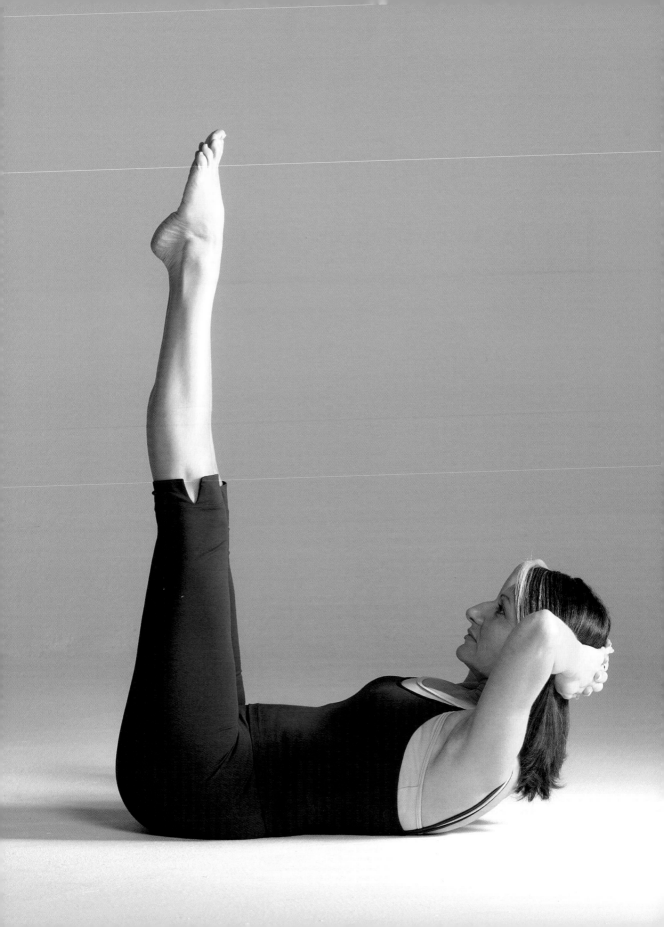

INTELLIGENT EXERCISE
WITH
PILATES & YOGA

LYNNE ROBINSON & HOWARD NAPPER
WITH CAROLINE BRIEN

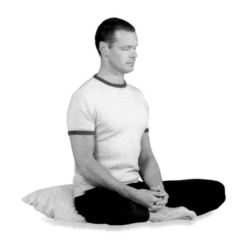

MACMILLAN

First published 2002 by Macmillan
an imprint of Pan Macmillan Ltd
Pan Macmillan, 20 New Wharf Road, London N1 9RR
Basingstoke and Oxford
Associated companies throughout the world
www.panmacmillan.com

ISBN 0 333 98952 X

Copyright © Lynne Robinson, Howard Napper
and Caroline Brien 2002

The right of Lynne Robinson, Howard Napper and Caroline Brien
to be identified as the authors of this work has been asserted by them
in accordance with the Copyright, Designs and Patents Act 1988.

Photography by Jim Marks except where otherwise indicated.
Technical illustrations by Raymond Turvey.

All rights reserved. No part of this publication may be
reproduced, stored in or introduced into a retrieval system, or
transmitted, in any form, or by any means (electronic, mechanical,
photocopying, recording or otherwise) without the prior written
permission of the publisher. Any person who does any unauthorized
act in relation to this publication may be liable to criminal
prosecution and civil claims for damages.

9 8 7 6 5 4 3 2 1

A CIP catalogue record for this book is available from
the British Library.

Typeset in Sabon by SX Composing DTP, Rayleigh, Essex
Printed and bound in Great Britain by Bath Press

Contents

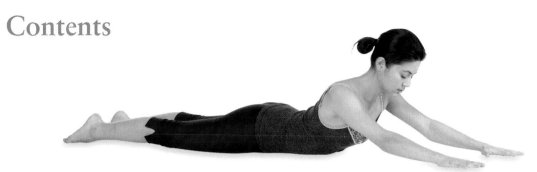

Acknowledgements

I have always been drawn towards gentler, more dignified, mindful types of exercise. The aerobics boom of the 1970s passed me by completely, in fact. I took up yoga in the 1980s, but sadly my inspiring yoga teacher, Shirley Lopez, went down with the *Herald of Free Enterprise* at Zeebrugge. I still miss Shirley and would like to think she would approve of this book. Working with Howard on this project has been an amazing experience, both personally and professionally. We have had so much fun! Thank you for sharing your knowledge with me (and the nation).

Caroline, you remained calm and collected and totally focused while Howard and I created chaos around you. Without you, this book would not have been written.

I am also extremely grateful for all the hard work and personal support that Gordon Wise, Charlie Mounter and, lately, Rafaela Romaya have put into this and all my books. I couldn't ask for more understanding publishers (for this, read: my next manuscript might be a few months late!).

Special thanks also to Jim Marks, our enormously talented photographer who was unbelievably patient and particularly creative, with both the camera and the scissors!

Last but by no means least, I wouldn't survive without the love and support of my family, Leigh, Rebecca and Emily.

Lynne Robinson

I would like to send my love and sincere thanks to my teacher John Stirk for the inspiration of yoga. Also to Francesca and my family for their love and constant support.

Howard Napper

My sincerest thanks to Lynne and Howard for asking me to be involved in this project – it's been an experience! As well as the wonderful team at Macmillan, I would like to add my gratitude to the fantastic Jim Marks for creative genius. Finally, much love to Justin and my family for their unwavering support and encouragement.

Caroline Brien

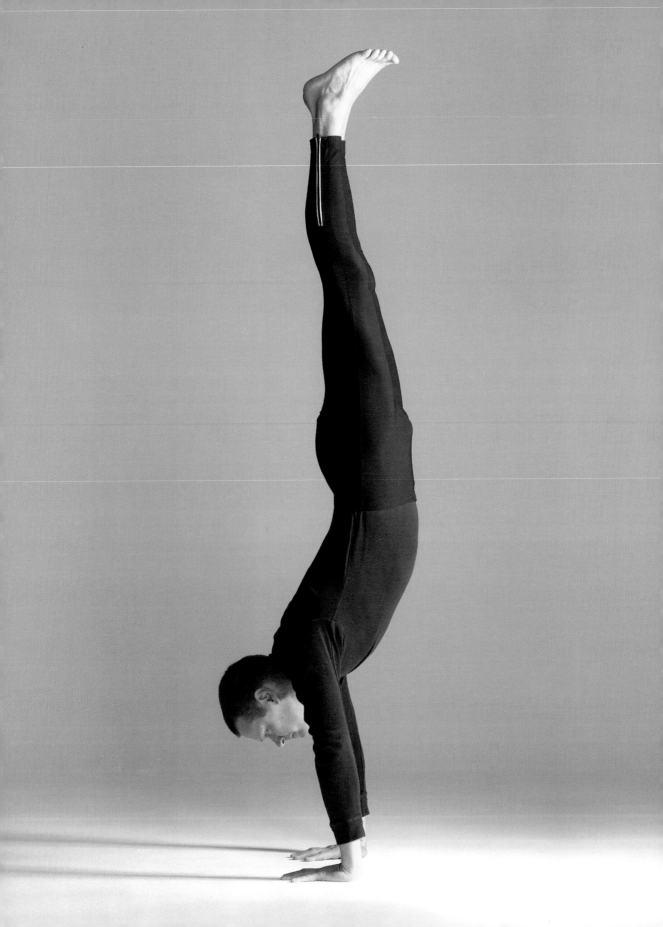

Pilates & yoga:

the perfect partners

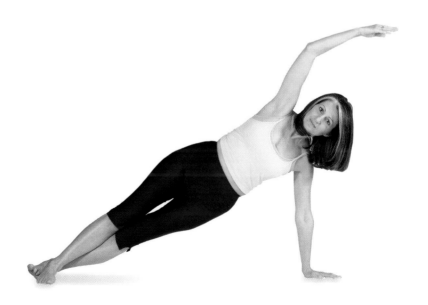

Two Disciplines, One Destination

Today, more people than ever are enjoying Pilates and yoga, thanks partly to the increasing desire for a more sophisticated approach to working the body. Most local gyms offer Pilates matwork classes and yoga classes, but it is seldom made clear that you don't have to choose one path or the other, you can do both. Because these two proven and established disciplines complement each other, we have created a programme that will give you a complete and enjoyable workout, using a varied combination of exercises.

When we got together to create this programme we discovered how much we had in common. Fundamental to both the Body Control Pilates® way of exercising and to the type of yoga described in this book, is that the original disciplines have been adapted to suit the needs of the modern body. Neither of us comes from a traditional fitness background or has classical training, but we have each developed a contemporary style through learning, practising and, ultimately, through teaching. It is these two individual styles (explained in more detail in the next chapter), which we have found can work in harmony to provide a balanced exercise programme.

Of course, there are differences in the way Pilates and yoga are practised, but our ultimate aim is to help people make sense of how they can work together. Rather than trying to fuse the two principles (after all, if you have good exercises, why change them?), we have looked for common ground to create a programme that explores the similarities and the reasons behind them, keeping the integrity of each. This is a great way to expand your exercise routine if you already practise either Pilates or yoga, but it also provides a sound introduction to a new way of exercising.

As you read this book and try the exercises in it, you will see just how alike Pilates and yoga are. Often, the movements are the same but the terminology is different, so wherever we can we use a common language. There will be areas where Pilates and yoga don't make a suitable marriage and make more sense when approached separately. This presents an opportunity to learn about your body, because the ability to choose is put into your hands. This choice is part of the concept of intelligent exercise.

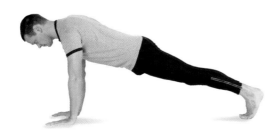
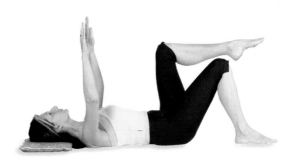

What Is Intelligent Exercise?

You will read a great deal in this book about intelligent exercise, but what exactly do we mean by it? The main thing that sets an intelligent approach to exercise apart from the outdated 'going for the burn' one is respect for the body at all times. Start with these five points to help you adopt this way of thinking:

- Not all knowledge is the right knowledge – it's up to you to find out who and where can offer you the best information (both industries suffer from bad or unqualified teachers, books and videos). Only the right practice makes perfect.
- Empower yourself by making your own decisions and taking responsibility for the exercises you do. That means practising too – after all, an hour of practice is worth many more hours of theory.
- Exercise is not about show, but how it feels from within. Don't worry about how you look in class or in front of a teacher – it's what you're *doing* that matters.
- Listen to your body and let what you feel govern how you proceed, rather than working through pain.
- Don't separate exercise from the rest of your life. There's no point finishing a great workout then feasting on unhealthy foods and slouching in an armchair – try to make it part of a balanced lifestyle.

Exercising intelligently also means recognizing and respecting both the similarities and differences between Pilates and yoga so that each time you exercise, you choose the path you want to follow. For example, some people find that the movement involved in Pilates helps concentrate the mind, while others enjoy the stillness of yoga. Both can help you find the same internal focus – it's really up to you. Remember that being in the moment is an important part of exercise. As the adage goes, don't miss the journey getting to the destination.

The best teacher is your body, so you can be your own teacher and your own pupil. That's not to say that you can't learn from others, but empower yourself by thinking into your body: use your judgement and experiment to find what's right for you. If you make sure you take the time to get the basic principles right, you'll reap the maximum benefits as you move through the programme. Done correctly, both Pilates and yoga will give you an amazing understanding and awareness of the body and how it works – done badly, there is a risk you may feel frustrated, develop bad habits and at worst, injure yourself.

Finally, don't think that the concept of intelligent exercise only applies to Pilates and yoga. You can take this approach to the gym, the swimming pool or the running track. It even applies to how you sit, eat and walk because it relates to every movement you make. Just remember to use your body intelligently!

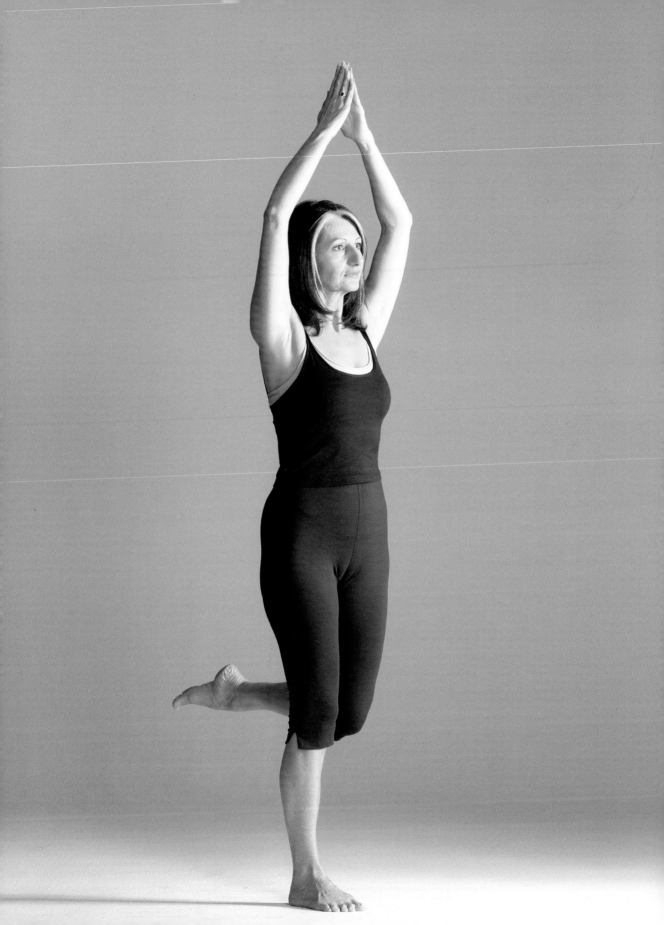

1 From past to present

Body Control Pilates® is based on the work of Joseph Pilates, who developed his method of body conditioning in the early decades of the twentieth century. Yoga has evolved from the wisdom of ancient Indian yogis. Common to both originators was an awareness of what they were doing with the body, but how appropriate is their wisdom in terms of today's fitness? This chapter will give you a better understanding of both disciplines, as well as explaining how each has been adapted to fit into this modern exercise programme.

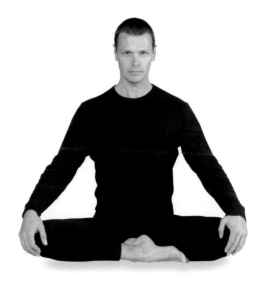

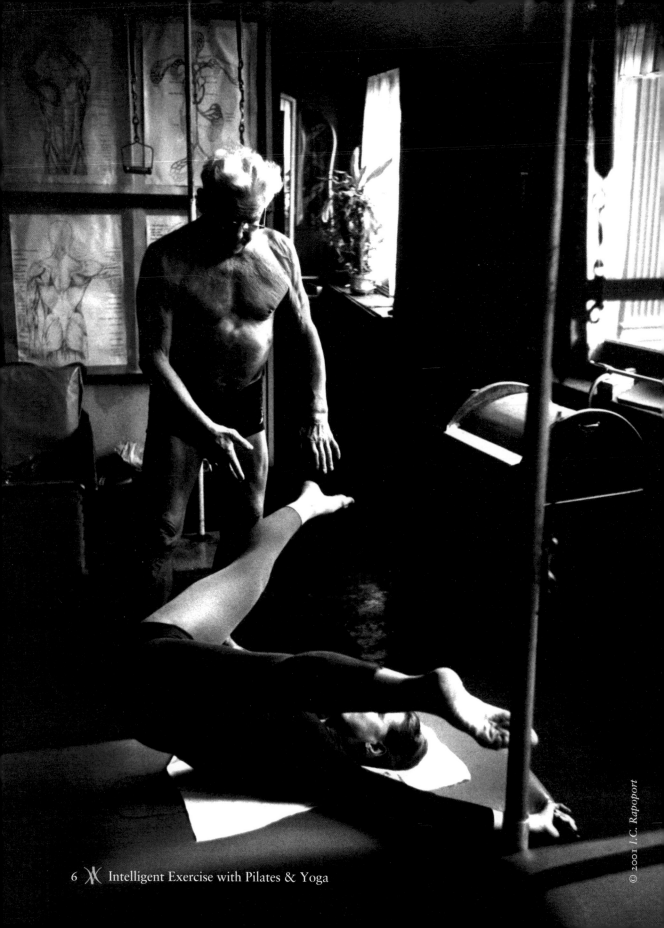

© 2001 I.C. Rapoport

Pilates Yesterday and Today (*Lynne Robinson*)

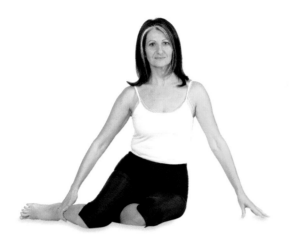

Pilates in the Past

Born in 1880 in Düsseldorf, Joseph Pilates was a sickly child who suffered from rickets, asthma and rheumatic fever. Determined to overcome his fragility, Joseph experimented with many different approaches to fitness rather than just following one established regime – something later reflected in his own teaching methods. Yoga, gymnastics, skiing, self-defence, dance, circus training and weight training all influenced him and by selecting the most effective aspects, he was able to work out a system that gave the body a perfect balance of strength and flexibility.

Proven on his own body, Joseph then began to apply these techniques to others. He was living in England when the First World War broke out, and his nationality caused him to be interned in Lancashire, and then on the Isle of Man. With time on his hands, Joseph helped in the camp infirmary and further developed his method by training fellow internees with amazing success. Many of these early trainees were war veterans with horrendous injuries, and much of Joseph's knowledge of rehabilitation came from this era.

At the end of the war, Joseph returned to Germany where he taught self-defence to the Hamburg police and the German army before emigrating to the United States in 1926. During the boat journey there, he met his future wife Clara. Realizing they shared the same views on fitness, the couple set up a studio together on Eighth Avenue in New York soon after their arrival. Joseph had a genius for designing exercise equipment to help rehabilitate his clients and develop the strength and flexibility they needed to perform his mat exercises. The studio attracted top ballet dancers, actors, gymnasts and athletes, all anxious to learn from him. The exercises described in Joseph's own books are very advanced, reflecting the professional nature of his studio clientele.

The Full Mat Programme he devised consisted of forty-plus choreographed mat exercises which were performed in a set order and which flowed one into the next comprising a total body conditioning workout. A hard taskmaster, one element that runs through his work is his insistence on commitment to the exercises – without excuse, they should be done regularly in order to realize results, making Pilates a discipline in more than one sense.

A fit and active eighty-six-year-old, Joseph Pilates died of smoke inhalation in 1967 following a fire at his studio.

Pilates Today

The true definition of Pilates is still being debated today. Joseph Pilates never took the initiative of setting up an official training programme and many of his disciples went on to teach their own versions of Pilates' method. But as Joseph rarely taught an exercise the same way twice (he geared his teaching to the needs of the individual and prescribed a unique programme to every client), each new teacher worked using a different emphasis. Hence today, you will find that there are many different levels of training (from two days to four years!) and many different ways of working.

There is however, a common philosophy at the root of all Pilates-based methods – it is less about *what* you do and more about *how* you do it. This has been a great advantage to Pilates teachers who have been able to absorb new ideas – from physiotherapy techniques and movement therapies for example – and incorporate them into the method without sacrificing its uniqueness. As a result, Pilates continues to evolve, moving forward without the constraint of a rigid set of rules.

In the last few years, the medical profession has also begun to look closely at why the method is so successful. Previously, many Pilates teachers taught intuitively, learning about good alignment and body use during their apprenticeship, though in many cases without fully knowing the technical medical terms for what they were doing. Under the close scrutiny of the medical establishment, the world of Pilates has had to re-examine its methods, and study precisely why they work so well.

The Pilates in This Book

As we have seen, Joseph Pilates devised a challenging matwork programme of about forty exercises, providing a total body workout. However, the majority of his clients were dancers who were better physically equipped to perform many of the difficult moves. This legacy can mean the average person may struggle with the movements and give up after the first class. I was introduced to Pilates by the wife of an osteopath who was treating me for a back injury and we quickly started to explore and learn from many different sources. We had to adapt the original exercises and create new ones quite simply because my body was not capable of doing the classical matwork.

Body Control Pilates® – the method used in this book – was set up in 1996 by Gordon Thomson and myself, and is based on the work of Joseph Pilates. It is unique in the way that it prepares the body for the classical exercises. Few people today could start their first session with the Hundred (see page 90), as was traditionally the case. We believe that you need to acquire the skills to perform such exercises gradually and this progressive approach has won the respect and support of leading medical bodies as well as top sports associations.

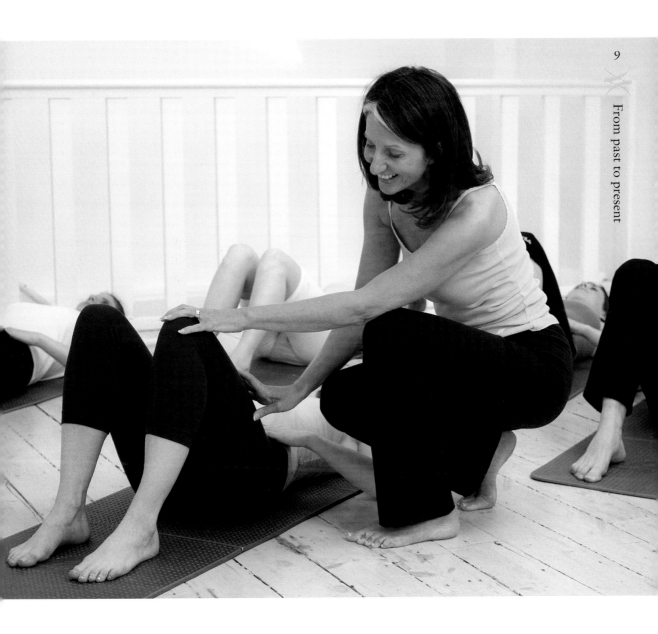

Yoga Yesterday and Today (*Howard Napper*)

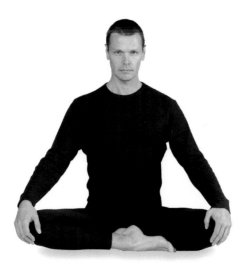

Yoga in the Past

Although some people might consider yoga just another trend, this 'trend' has been around for between three to five thousand years. In fact, one of the things that attracted me to yoga was that it has its roots in an ancient tradition. No one is exactly sure when or where yoga began, but documents dating back as early as 2,700 BC depict figures seated in yoga positions. In these early years, the word yoga was associated with the Hindu tradition of spiritual discipline and involved control over the mind through prolonged periods of meditation. Although the various techniques may have differed, the goal was the same: self-realization or enlightenment.

There is a wide range of translations for the word yoga, but the most commonly accepted is yoke or union. It can be found in classical Hindu literature such as the *Upanishad*, which dates back to the second millennium BC, as well

as the *Bhagavad Gita*, which dates back to the third or fourth century BC. However, it wasn't until the *Yoga Sutras* of Patanjali, which compiled existing knowledge of yoga philosophy some time around the second century BC, that it became systematized.

The *Yoga Sutras* consist of an eight-limbed pathway. The pathway begins with two codes of conduct, called yama (general ethical principles) and niyama (self-restraint). It continues with: asana (postures); pranayama (breath control); pratyahara (withdrawal of the senses); dharana (concentration); dhyana (meditation); and, finally, samadhi (ecstasy), a self-realized state of being. Of these eight limbs, only asana dealt with the purely physical side of yoga and is the one that most people associate with it today. The word asana itself derives from the Sanskrit for seat or, more generally, the place or manner in which a yogi sits. Over time, asana has come to mean posture, and these postures – or positions – were used to help the yogis maintain their bodies in order to sit in meditation for prolonged periods of time. According to Patanjali, they were to be 'steady and comfortable'. This is achieved through correct alignment of the body, which gives stability and relaxation. In turn, the alignment opens and frees the body, allowing prana (energy) to move along its axis – the spine.

The word prana is used often in yoga and is understood as energy or life force, but its true meaning comes from two Sanskrit words, derived from 'pra' meaning constant and 'na' meaning movement. In freeing the body from tension – which is only blocked energy – we allow constant movement, or waves of energy

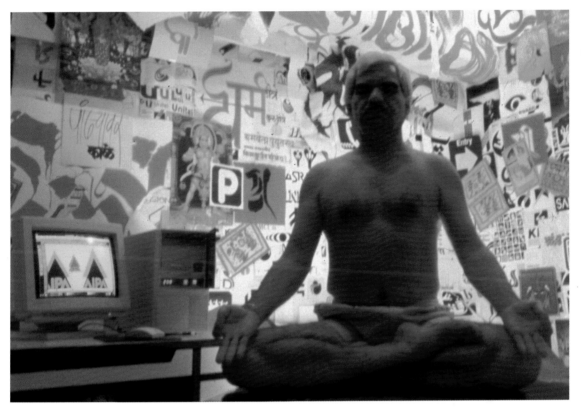

Mr Sudarshan Dheer, meditation yoga, India. *Private Collection / Bridgeman Art Library*

to flow uninhibited. One of the main ways of achieving this is through the breath and one of Patanjali's other eight limbs – pranayama – dealt specifically with the art and science of the breath. The asana postures and pranayama are closely linked: each asana is underpinned by pranayama, awareness of the breath.

As the practice of asana evolved, it acquired a therapeutic function that in turn led to the construction of more and more sophisticated asanas. This led to the development of Hatha yoga. The direct translation of hatha is force, although this is somewhat misleading. In his book *Light on Yoga*, contemporary Hatha yoga master B. K. S. Iyengar describes hatha as force, but then goes on to say, '. . . it is so-called because it prescribes rigorous discipline, in order to find union with the supreme'. The word hatha also has its roots in the words 'ha', meaning sun and 'tha', meaning moon. Hatha can therefore be understood to mean the union between the sun and the moon, or the joining of male and female energies, yin and yang, positive and negative. Hatha yoga implies the coming together of any set of polarities in order to find transcendence. Yoga is a union between mind and body, which leads to a transcendent state of being known as jiva-mukta – liberated soul or supreme spirit.

Yoga Today

The idea of union is a major theme in Vedic philosophy. The great Indian philosopher J. Krishnamurti wrote, 'Where there is separation there is inevitably conflict.' This echoes the yogic belief that everything in the universe is ultimately one – very different from our Western traditions of thought, which emphasize a fundamental split in the self: the separation between mind and body. Primacy is usually given to the mind, or thought; the body is seen as something separate, something to be conquered and overcome. So when yoga moved to the West, no wonder it was met with some confusion.

The ground for its introduction here was laid in 1893, with the arrival from India of Swami Vivekananda, who gained recognition when he represented Hinduism at the World Parliament of Religions in Chicago. Soon after this, the West's awareness of Indian philosophy began to grow through the work of groups such as the Theosophical Society, founded in America by Madame Blavatsky. Members of the society included some of the most prominent intellectuals of the day, for example, Aldous Huxley, Frank Lloyd Wright and W. B. Yeats. The Theosophical Society arranged for most of the ancient Indian philosophical texts available at the time to be translated, including the *Yoga Sutras* of Patanjali, which were interpreted by English novelist and Theosophical Society member, Christopher Isherwood.

Over the next few decades, the West's interest in Indian philosophy continued to grow. The teaching of J. Krishnamurti considerably widened the appeal and understanding of Vedic philosophy. With an increasing awareness of the philosophy grew an interest in the physical practice with which it was so closely linked – yoga. In 1935, the eminent Swiss psychologist Carl G. Jung described yoga as, 'one of the greatest things the human mind has ever created'. But it wasn't until the 1950s that an interest in Hatha yoga really emerged through the work of teachers such as B. K. S. Iyengar, who taught both Europeans and Americans. One of his most renowned pupils was the violinist Yehudi Menuhin, who wrote the foreword for Iyengar's book, *Light on Yoga*. By the time of its publication in 1966, groups people throughout the West were practising Hatha yoga.

It wasn't long before people from all over the world were travelling to India to discover yoga and the Vedic philosophy from which it emerged. Then, following the Beatles' journey to India in 1968 to study transcendental meditation with their guru Marharishi Mahesh Yogi, all that was Indian firmly became part of the hippy culture. Through the seventies and eighties, Hatha yoga continued to have a healthy following in the West, although the people who practised it were generally considered to be a bit odd or simply old hippies. This changed in the mid-nineties when people started to become bored with the mindless 'no pain, no gain' gym culture and a little-known style of Hatha yoga called Astanga, came to the fore. Astanga fitted in perfectly with the new mantra of 'perfect body, perfect mind', and was endorsed by celebrities such as Sting and Madonna. Soon it was estimated that there were more people doing yoga in California than in all of India!

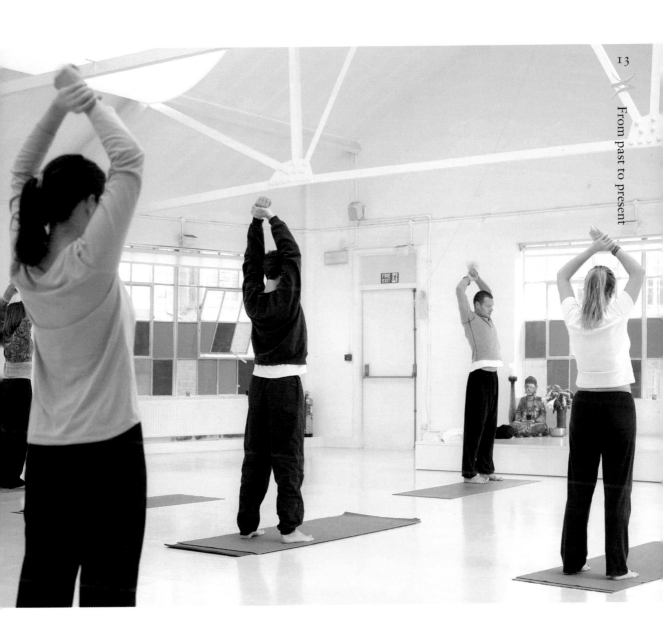

According to *Time* magazine, there are around fifteen million people practising yoga in America today; there is probably an equivalent number practising in Europe. So a centuries old discipline that started out preparing yogis to sit for long periods of time in meditation, today finds a place in a society where people may require help with sitting for long periods of time in front of a computer.

The Yoga in This Book

Many different types of yoga have emerged over its long history so to say that any one particular style is representational of all types is impossible. Although I have studied many different types of yoga, the one I talk about in this book is the one I love and know best.

I was particularly drawn by the awareness and sensitivity that this type of yoga brings to the body – qualities that probably came about because a woman devised it. She was an Italian named Vanda Scaravelli and one of her main aims was that of self-empowerment – constantly listening to and trusting the inherent intelligence of one's own body. Her teachings centre around three main themes: the spine, gravity and the breath, and how they relate to each other. She was fortunate enough to have had the opportunity to befriend and study with two of the great yoga teachers of our time: B. K. S. Iyengar, from whom she learned the importance of correct alignment, and T. K. V. Desikachar, who showed her the value of the breath in each position. She was also greatly influenced by her friend J. Krishnamurti, who spoke of the worth of being one's own teacher and one's own pupil, empowered to be able to listen to an inner wisdom.

Vanda Scaravelli died in 1999, aged ninety-one. At the age of eighty-three, however, she wrote her inspiring book *Awakening the Spine* (available in paperback, 1991, Harper San Francisco). In it, she is seen demonstrating some of the most advanced forms of yoga with complete openness in the body. Although she never wanted her type of yoga to have a label or be named after her, because of our need to label almost everything it has become known as Scaravelli yoga. Sadly, I never had the opportunity to work with Vanda, but discovered her work through a wonderful Hatha yoga teacher called John Stirk. John changed my yoga immensely and in doing so he also changed my life. He worked with Vanda for many years and this, combined with an amazing knowledge of the body gained from his background as a top osteopath, made him the ideal person to pass on the unique and subtle principles of her deep yoga.

Vanda Scaravelli/Rob Howard

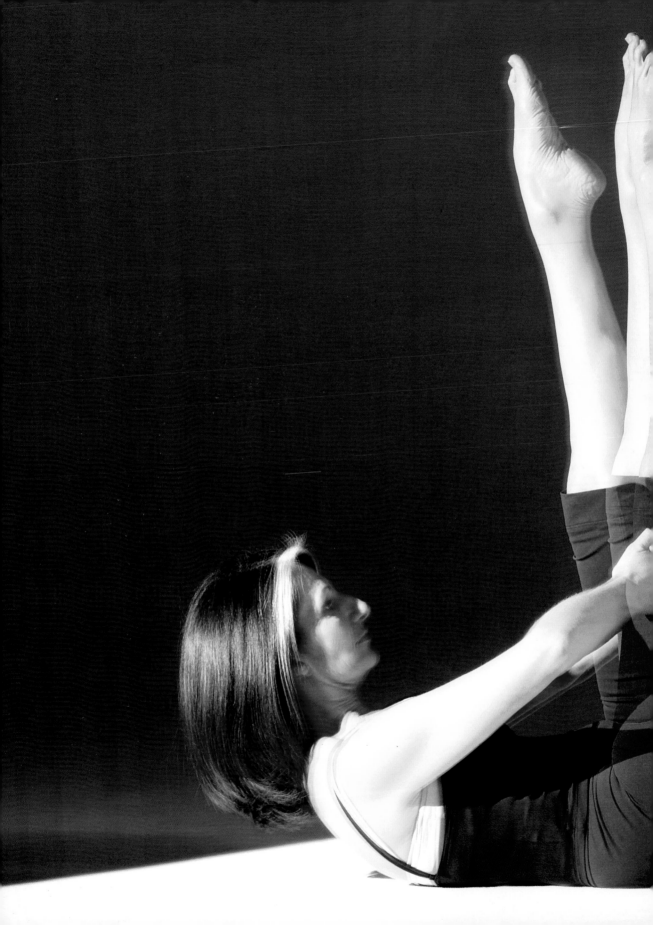

2 Behind the programme

This chapter deals with the key principles and theory behind Pilates and yoga. It is the ideal way to prepare for exercising intelligently as it explains how and why each movement is done in a particular way. In order to do this, it is necessary to look first at the body's capabilities.

The Principles of the Body

Whichever sport or form of exercise you are doing
– be it Pilates, yoga, tennis or gym work – the same
fundamental principles apply to your body.

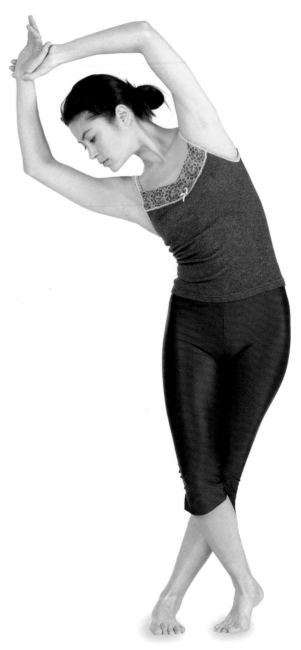

Natural Flowing Movement

Watch any healthy children play and you will see that they move easily and freely, without inhibition or restriction – in other words, with natural flowing movements. Their bodies have grace, strength, stamina, speed and flexibility. Adults, however, form habits, constantly repeating the same movements every day, and diminishing the body's ability to make these childlike motions. If you don't use it, you lose it!

There are three elements that make up the body's movement:

- nervous system – control
- skeletal structure – bones, joints, ligaments, cartilage
- musculature

Movement depends on messages to and from the brain via the nervous system – constant input and output – and what has come to the fore in medical research is the importance of good input. Because the brain remembers patterns of movement rather than individual muscle contractions, repeating correct patterns locks them into the muscle memory bank.

This begins to explain why the body loses its natural flowing movement with age. That freedom is best evident in children up to five years old, when they first enter the classroom and start to spend hours sitting on chairs in front of desks for most of the week. At home there are more chairs – for watching television and playing computer games. As young adults, they face piles of homework and exams, until inevitably, stress levels rise. They carry heavily loaded backpacks over one shoulder distorting the spine and musculature and, on reaching

puberty, their bodies change again. To make things worse, good posture does not seem to be fashionable among teenagers – slouching is much more hip! When they are older and go to work, the chances are they will still sit at a desk all day before driving home to slump on the couch all evening. All the natural flowing movements used as a child are now restricted to a limited range of repetitive actions.

Muscle is dependent upon, and reflects, patterns of use. Disuse or misuse of muscles are associated with changes in their function. By not using them, you particularly affect the anti-gravity postural muscles that lie deep within the body. It is these muscles that support (or stabilize) the spine and other joints. If they weaken, other muscles will take on their role and muscle imbalances will occur.

The key therefore to reversing years of bad body use is to start from scratch – slowly re-learning and re-educating the body to move correctly again. The nervous system is incredibly adaptable and will reorganize itself as a result of training. There are three stages to this process:

- thinking about good movement
- practising good movement
- automatic 'grooved' movement, which becomes a muscle memory (an engram)

The exercise in this book will take you through the stages needed to change your existing movement patterns, ensuring that every action is performed correctly to restore natural flowing movement.

Muscles and Movement

Muscles, the active part of the equation, work together in groups to move our bones. Working as a team, one muscle may act as the main mover (agonist); the opposing muscles allow the movement to take place (antagonist); other muscles set the bones in the correct position (stabilizers) or add slight variation (synergists). With everything working correctly and in the right order, you have a good pattern of use – a sound recruitment pattern – and normal movement.

Top right: Multifidus. As you 'zip up and hollow' multifidus is engaged, stabilizing your lumbar spine.

Below: Transversus Abdominis (your girdle of strength)

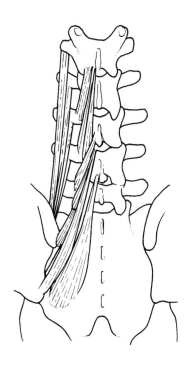

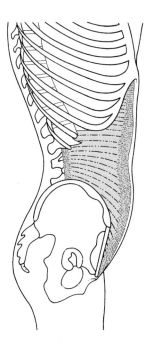

The importance of the stabilizing muscles is becoming increasingly clear in medical research. If you want to take a book from a high shelf, for example, it is not the hand or shoulder muscles that are engaged first, but the deep postural muscles which stabilize the lumbar spine, ensuring that one vertebra doesn't shear too far off its neighbour. These muscles are transversus abdominis and a deep back muscle called multifidus. They engage to form a natural corset or girdle of strength around the centre of the body so that movement can take place easily, smoothly and safely. This stable base is essential to the body in the same way that a tower crane needs a stable base while its long arm moves around. Likewise, problems can arise when these deep stabilizing muscles are not working correctly, for example, if the body is out of alignment and holds an incorrect position for any length of time. When stabilizing muscles are held stretched, they weaken, forcing other muscles to take over the stabilizing role – the wrong muscles are then doing the wrong job. This is the birth of a faulty recruitment pattern. In order for a muscle to work efficiently, it needs to be at its optimal length. When it is held over-stretched or over-lengthened, it cannot work effectively; neither will it work properly if it is over-shortened.

Simply speaking, muscles have two types of role: a stabilizing role that holds bones in place and a mobilizing role that creates large movements. In an ideal world, muscles designed to stabilize will stabilize, and those designed to mobilize will mobilize. Returning to the image of the crane, the stabilizers are the stable base, while the mobilizers make the large sweeping movements of the arm. These two types of muscles have different characteristics. Stabilizing muscles have to work for long periods of time – they have to hold tone and need endurance, are often shorter in length and usually lie deeper within the body. They should be worked at below 20 per cent of their full efficiency. Mobilizing muscles, on the other hand, make big movements, such as moving the limbs around. In order to make these movements they work in phases, turning on and off. They also tend to be more superficial, lying closer to the surface of the body and are usually quite long. Mobilizers fatigue quickly and work at between 40 to 100 per cent of their full efficiency.

Some muscles work as stabilizers in some movements and mobilizers in others. If, however, a deep stabilizing muscle is not functioning properly due to weakness, a mobilizer may take on a stabilizing role which, with time, changes its fibre type so that it will no longer be able to work efficiently as a mobilizer. For example, your hamstring muscles, which for many movements act as mobilizing muscles making larger movements, are often obliged to stabilize the pelvis because the deep gluteals (buttocks) are too weak. Consequently, they tighten and shorten. No amount of stretching will lengthen them while they have to keep stabilizing. The solution to this problem would be to strengthen the deep gluteals so that the hamstrings can let go.

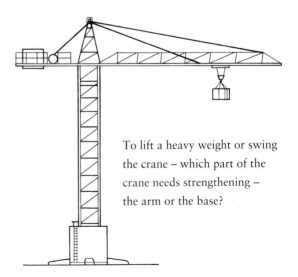

To lift a heavy weight or swing the crane – which part of the crane needs strengthening – the arm or the base?

The main stabilizers

The Pilates and yoga exercises in this book are
designed to ensure that the body uses the
muscles correctly. The detailed directions given
about the position of your pelvis, shoulders,
breathing and abdominal muscles mean that
you will know what you are doing as you move,
automatically engaging the right muscles and
letting the rest follow.

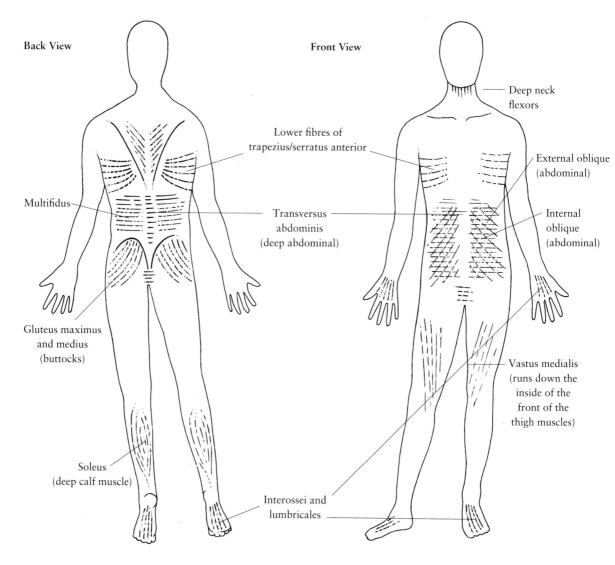

Back View

Front View

Deep neck
flexors

Lower fibres of
trapezius/serratus anterior

External oblique
(abdominal)

Multifidus

Transversus
abdominis
(deep abdominal)

Internal
oblique
(abdominal)

Gluteus maximus
and medius
(buttocks)

Vastus medialis
(runs down the
inside of the
front of the
thigh muscles)

Soleus
(deep calf muscle)

Interossei and
lumbricales

The Principles and Theory of Pilates

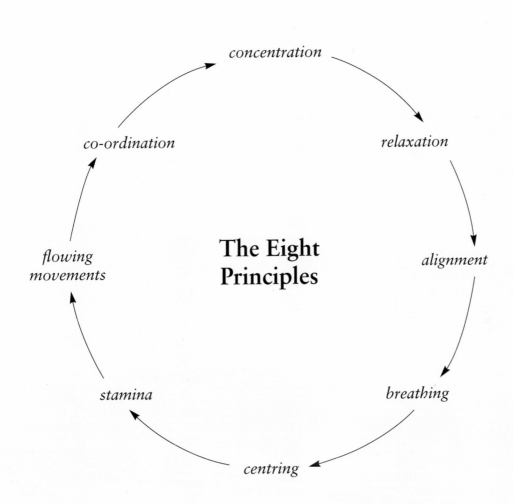

Relaxation

This is the starting point for everyone learning Pilates. It may seem a strange way to begin an exercise routine, but the first priority is to ensure that every day stress isn't brought into a session. Learning how to recognize and release areas of unwanted tension is essential before you workout, as it helps prevent the use of the wrong muscles. We need to learn how to switch off over-dominant muscles otherwise they will continue to overwork, perpetuating unsound movement patterns. Most people hold tension in the back of the neck and upper shoulders, but when a lot of time is spent sitting, the muscles around the front of the hips, the low back and the hamstrings, become very tight too.

The Relaxation Position on page 48 is a good way to start a session – you will also notice that we use it as the starting and finishing position for many of the exercises. As you advance in Pilates however, you should be able to use any simple exercise to the same effect. Please note that by relaxation we do not mean collapse, but a release of unnecessary tension in readiness to move.

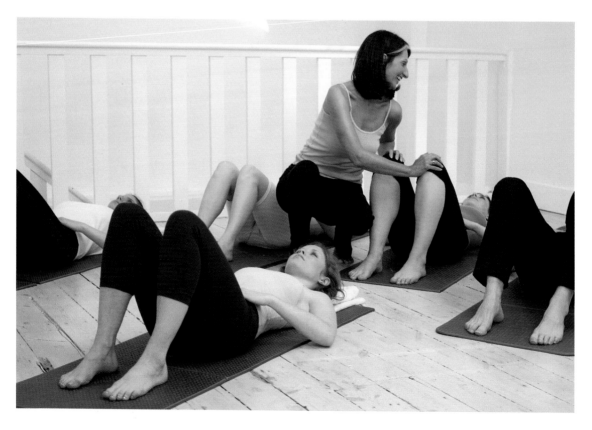

Concentration

Another benefit that comes with relaxation
is focus. Pilates is a mental and physical
conditioning programme that should train both
mind and body. It requires you to focus on each
movement made and develops your body's
sensory feedback or kinaesthetic sense, so that
you know where you are in space and what
you are doing with every part of your body.
Although the movements themselves may
become automatic with time, you still have
to concentrate because there is always a
further level of awareness to achieve. These
proprioceptive awareness skills are vital
to good movement and can be applied
to other activities.

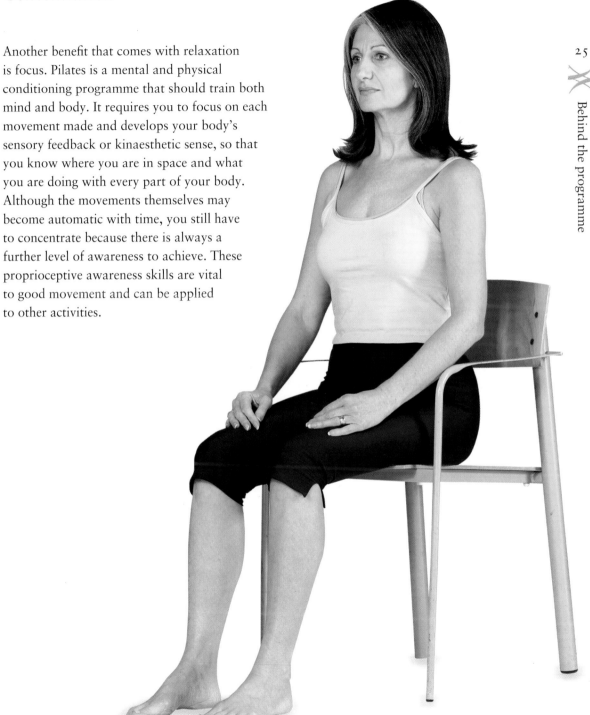

Alignment

By constantly reminding the body of how it should be standing, sitting or lying and by moving correctly, you can bring the body into better alignment – essential to restore muscle balance in the body. If you exercise without due attention to the correct position of the joints, you risk stressing them as well as building imbalance into the surrounding muscles. Good alignment of each and every part of the body while exercising is crucial.

The checklist (right) should help you align your body correctly.

The Compass on page 49 is designed to help you find the correct neutral position of the pelvis and the spine. Once you are familiar with this in the Relaxation Position, you should practise finding neutral while standing, sitting and lying on your side so that it becomes normal. All the exercises should be performed in this neutral position unless otherwise specified. Please note that, occasionally, if the muscles around the pelvis are very out of balance, you may find neutral difficult to maintain. When this is the case, consult a qualified Pilates practitioner, as it is often necessary to work in what is the best neutral you can achieve. After a few months, as the muscles begin to rebalance, achieving neutral ought to feel more comfortable.

Start at the base of your feet:

- Lengthen upwards through the spine and the top of your head.
- Allow your neck to release.
- Relax your shoulder blades down into your back.
- Keep your breastbone soft.
- Keep your elbows open.
- Keep the natural curves of your spine.
- Have your head, ribcage and pelvis balanced on top of each other.
- Check that the pelvis is in neutral (see page 49).
- When you bend your knees for an exercise they should be directly over the centre of each foot.
- Stand with the feet hip-distance apart and with the legs parallel.
- Keep the weight even on both feet – do not allow them to roll in or out.

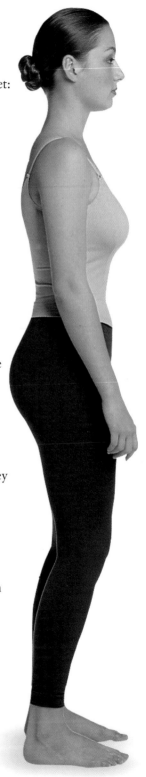

Breathing

As you can help or hinder a movement by breathing, all Pilates exercises are carefully created to reinforce and encourage the right muscle recruitment by correct breathing and timing of the breath.

Stand in front of a mirror and watch as you take a deep breath. Do your shoulders rise up around the ears? Perhaps your lower stomach expands when you breathe in? Most of us breathe inefficiently. Ideally, you should breathe in wide and full into your back and sides. This makes sense because the lungs are situated in the ribcage and by expanding it, the volume of the cavity is increased and the capacity for oxygen intake is therefore increased too. It also encourages maximum use of the lower part of the lungs.

This type of breathing – called thoracic or lateral breathing – makes the upper body more fluid and mobile. The lungs become like bellows, with the lower ribcage expanding wide as you breathe in and closing down as you breathe out. You shouldn't block the descent of the diaphragm but should encourage the movement to be widthways and into the back. The exercise on page 45 will help you to breathe laterally. As important to Pilates is the timing of the breath. Most people find this difficult at first, especially if you are used to other fitness regimes, but once you have mastered it, it makes sense.

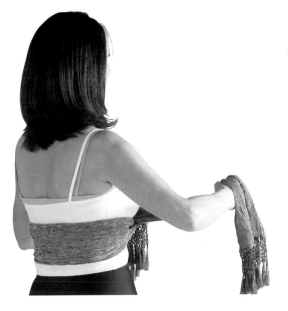

As a general rule:

- Breathe in to prepare for a movement (zipped and hollowed).
- Breathe out, with a strong centre to protect the spine and move (still zipped).
- Breathe in to recover.

Moving on the exhalation will enable you to relax into the stretch and prevent you from tensing. It also offers greater core stability at the hardest part of the exercise and safeguards against holding the breath, which can unduly stress the heart and lead to serious complications.

Centring: Creating a Girdle of Strength

Joseph Pilates discovered that if he hollowed his navel back towards his spine, the lower back felt protected. He had no knowledge of core stability or transversus abdominis, but had developed superb body awareness and thus introduced the direction 'navel to spine' into all his exercises. Modern medical research confirms that the best stability comes when the action begins with the pelvic floor and then engages the lower abdominals. This is why the direction 'zip up and hollow' is used in Body Control Pilates®. As you breathe out, draw up the muscles of the pelvic floor and hollow the lower abdominals back to the spine as if you are doing up an internal zip. Then hold the zip while you breathe normally.

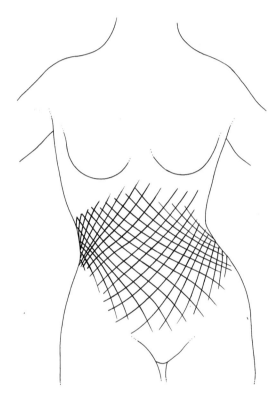

You will notice that the word 'hollow' is used to describe the action. It is very important that you do not grip your abdominals tightly as this creates unnecessary tension as well as usually engaging the wrong muscles. Remember that stabilizing muscles need to be worked at less than 20 per cent of their full effort.

Once you have learned to create a strong centre, add movements. The exercises starting on page 56 will take you through this step by step.

Co-ordination

You should now be ready to add movements
such as rotation, flexion and extension to the
equation while maintaining a strong centre.
Initially this isn't easy, but it soon becomes
an automatic (grooved) movement – a muscle
memory. Meanwhile, the actual process of
learning this co-ordination is excellent mental
and physical training, stimulating the two-way
communication channel to feed the brain good
movement and sound recruitment patterns.
Start with small motions and build up to more
complicated combinations – the idea is to be
constantly challenged. However, no matter
what exercise you are performing, the
movements must be correctly executed, with
the right alignment and breathing and the right
muscles doing the work. Repetition of these
sound movement patterns will start to change
the way you move for the better.

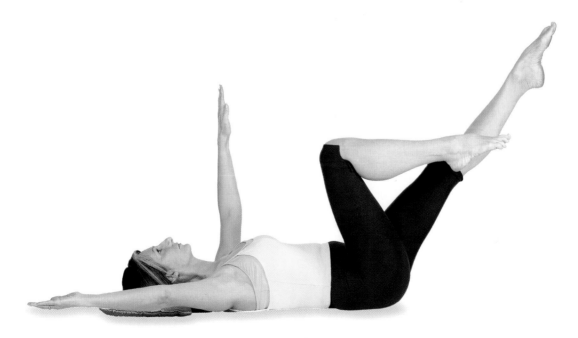

Flowing Movements

Pilates is all about natural flowing movements
performed correctly, gracefully and with
control. You will not be required to twist into
awkward positions or to strain. The movements
are generally slow, lengthening away from a
strong centre, which gives you the opportunity
to check alignment and focus on using the right
muscles. Slow doesn't mean easy though – in
fact it is harder to do an exercise slowly than
quickly and it is also less easy to cheat!

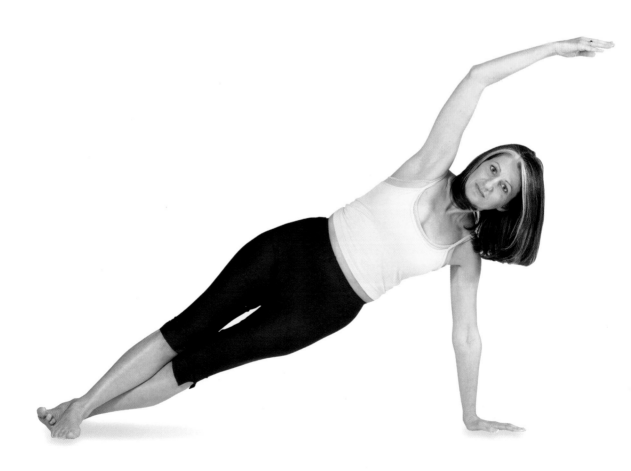

Stamina

Finally, we wish to build endurance and stamina into the body. We can do this by challenging stability, working with longer levers (for example, an extended leg rather than a bent one), adding load with weights, using resistance or unstable surfaces. Many people will complain of tiredness after a day on their feet, simply because standing badly is tiring: the ribcage is compressed and as a consequence, the lungs are constricted. As you learn to open and lengthen the body, breathing becomes more efficient. All Pilates exercises are designed to encourage the respiratory, lymphatic and circulatory systems to function more effectively.

When you become more proficient at the exercises, and your muscles begin to work correctly, you will discover that your overall stamina improves dramatically. You will no longer be wasting energy holding on to unnecessary tension or moving inefficiently. Think of a well-serviced car where the engine is tuned and the wheels aligned – it runs more efficiently, as will your body.

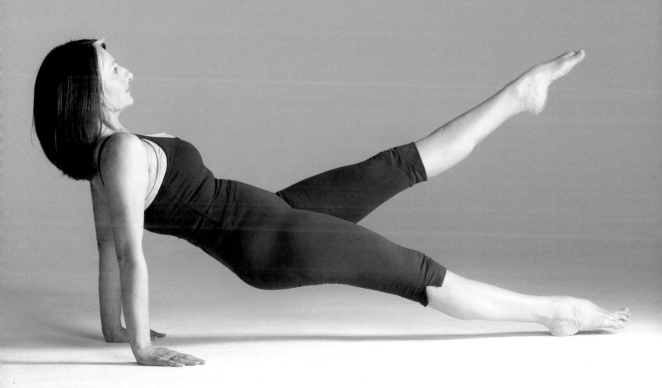

The Principles and Theory of Yoga

The principles of yoga usually refer to the eight limbs laid out by Patanjali (see Yoga in the Past page 10). These were aids on the path that the ancient yogi would take towards self-realization and, although still practised today, they are not immediately relevant to the yoga you will be practising. The focus is on a different set of principles – those that relate to the Vanda Scaravelli style of yoga.

You will recall that Vanda distilled the principles of her yoga down to three:

- Breath – follow the movement of the breath through the entire body.
- Gravity – be aware of aligning the body with the gravitational pull as well as releasing superficial tension.
- The spine – keep the spine supple and allow it to open out in two directions from the area around the navel.

These principles of the breath, gravity and the spine all have to do with developing a sense of inner awareness – the very thing that makes yoga unique. Most forms of exercise or sport are concerned with external movement or movement through space but yoga, by contrast, is concerned with internal movement. When you learn to listen to the body – to know and accept it rather than resisting it – you will realize that what you may take to be stillness is in fact an extraordinary dynamism: a subtle internal wave rolls ceaselessly along the spine in response to gravity and the breath. Awareness of this movement gives insight into the internal and universal dance that flows through all of us and is the source of an immense power.

Breath

In yoga, the breath is known as prana and as mentioned already, there is a whole practice devoted to working with the breath called pranayama. Most cultures acknowledge the importance of the breath in some way: prana is the same as 'chi' in China; while in the West we know it as 'life force'. In fact, the word 'spirit' comes from the Latin *spiritus*, meaning 'the breath of life'.

Breathing draws oxygen into every cell of the body. It is a nourishing function, bringing energy. In addition, the breath is also a movement and it is the awareness of this movement that can bring inward focus. This is the first step to connecting mind and body – it is nothing more than being present and mindful of our own physicality. Once you are able to be mindful of the breath, you can use this mindfulness to connect to other parts of the body – be it a shoulder blade or a deep muscle within the hip.

Ultimately, as you start to breathe fully and mindfully, the breath no longer just relates to the lungs. The whole of the body starts to become part of the respiratory system and from head to toe, expands and contracts with wave after wave of inhalation and exhalation.

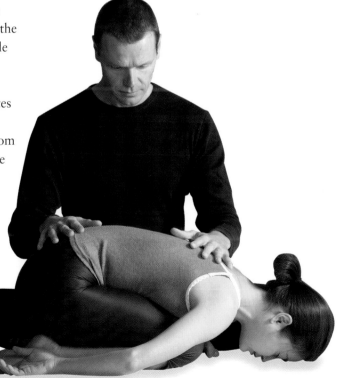

Gravity

Gravity, along with the breath, is one of the fundamental constants of life. Both are present from the moment of birth until death and therefore little attention is paid to their moment to moment effect on the body. But gravity is a powerful and extraordinary force that keeps the whole of the universe together. Likewise, for the body to function efficiently, it has to work with gravity rather than against it.

Work with gravity by yielding to it – not in the sense of collapsing, but by giving way to the gravitational pull while still retaining the integrity of the body's alignment. When this happens, not only is gravity able to pull the body, but it is able to lift it as well. Just like the rebound of a bouncing ball, elasticity in our core allows us to be open to both gravity and levity. However, holding tension in the body will prevent the yielding and in turn block levity, reflecting the need for a strong but supple core. The more elasticity the body has, the more lift or levity it will gain.

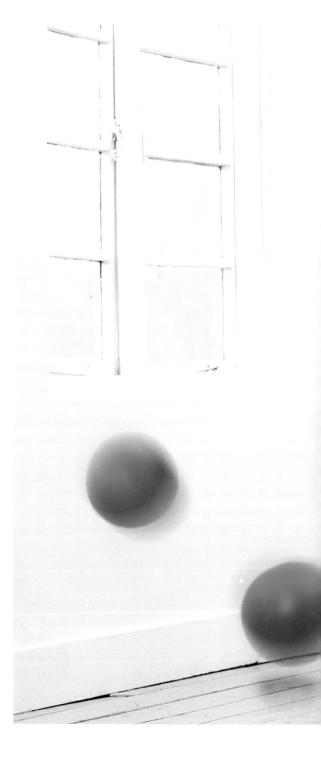

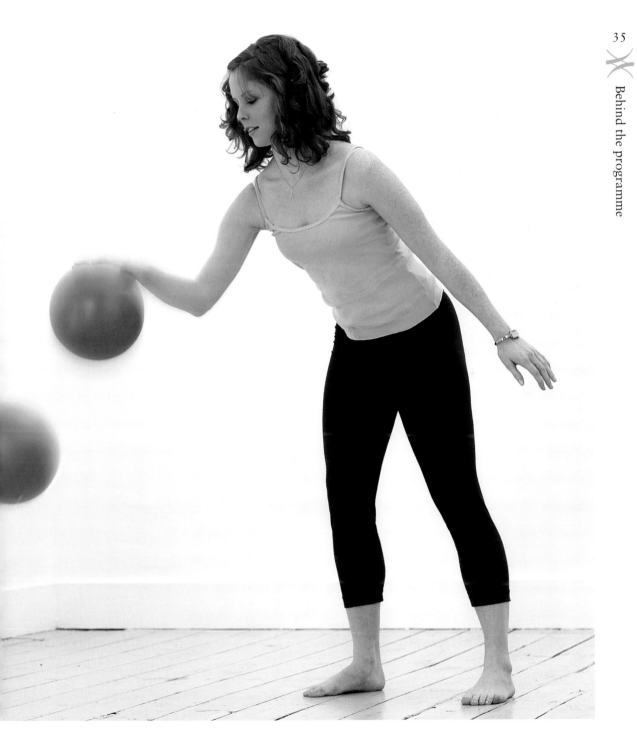

The Spine

The human spine has evolved in such a way that gravity falls straight through it. It is made up of four opposing curves, which counterbalance each other, allowing us to stand upright and move freely while giving optimum support to the head. An interconnected series of muscles, known as anti-gravity postural muscles, help to hold the spine in place. In supporting the spine along with the ligaments, these muscles give stability as well as creating lift. All movement begins with these deep muscles.

In addition to being important for movement, the spine houses the life-sustaining central nervous system. Think of this as the tail of the brain that branches out to all the muscles and internal organs in the body, controlling sensation, overall well-being and movement. If the spine becomes compressed, jammed or sleepy, it can compromise the nervous system's ability to operate efficiently, but as you awaken and create openness in the spine, you will invigorate the nervous system, allowing more information to move to and from the brain and the rest of the body.

If the spine is the core of the body, then the centre – the area around the navel – is its seed. Like a plant whose roots and stem grow in opposite directions, the body opens out from the centre, rooting as well as naturally lifting. Once you realize this, you no longer have to push up from the feet to lengthen the body. Instead you will find that as you breathe out, the spine itself is capable of elongating. The exhalation moves the lungs, diaphragm and abdomen all back in the direction of the spine, releasing the deep muscles that hold it in place and allowing it to lengthen. As you breathe in, the reverse happens and the spine contracts. This is an involuntary movement that cannot be forced. You can only begin to feel this deep movement once you start to release excess tension, allowing the whole body to respond to the breath like an accordion.

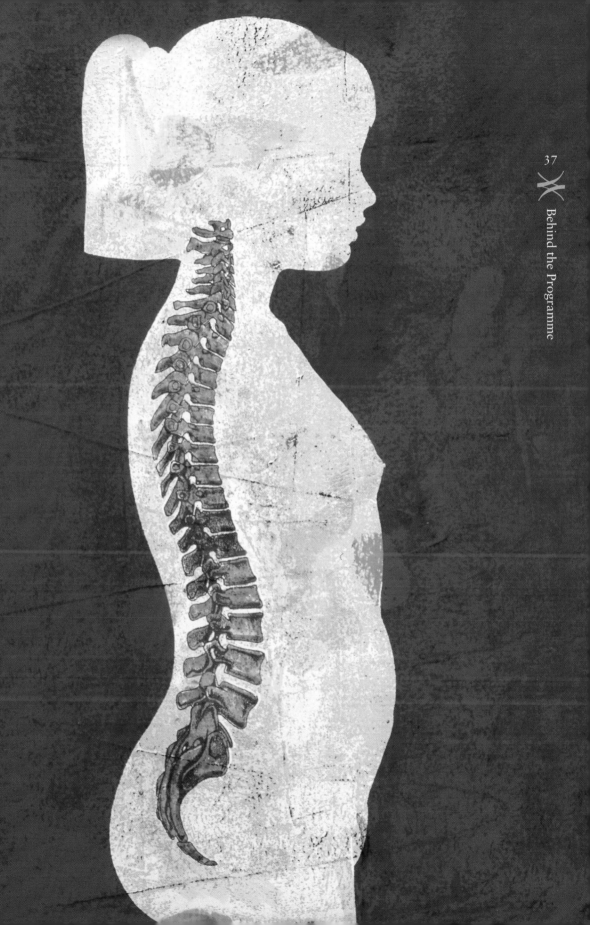

Hans-Ulrich Osterwalder / Science Photo Library

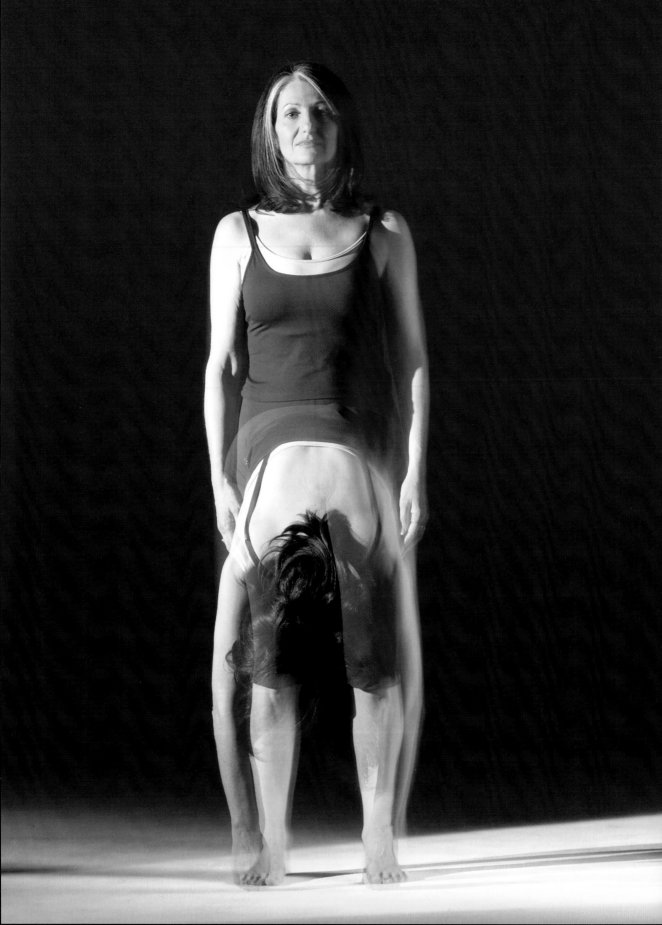

3 Preparing to exercise

How to Prepare

What You Need:

- a padded, non-slip mat or a yoga mat folded in half
- a folded towel or small, flat pillow
- a plump pillow
- a flatter, bedroom pillow
- a tennis ball
- a yoga belt or a dressing-gown belt
- loose, comfortable clothing and bare feet

Before You Begin

Prepare the space you are going to exercise in by making it warm, comfortable and free from distractions. Please do not exercise if:

- You are feeling unwell.
- You have just eaten a heavy meal.
- You have been drinking alcohol.
- You are in pain from an injury. Always consult your practitioner first, as rest may be needed before exercise.
- You have been taking painkillers, as they will mask any warning signs.
- You are undergoing medical treatment or are taking drugs. Again, you will need to consult your practitioner first.

Remember, it is always wise to consult your doctor before taking up a new exercise regime. For example, many of the exercises are wonderful for back-related problems, but you should always seek expert guidance first. *Please also note that not all the exercises in this programme are suitable for use during pregnancy.*

How to Use This Book

This programme has been put together so that it is straightforward, methodical and dynamic. We have used a key to indicate if the exercise comes from Pilates (*p*), yoga (*y*) or both (*p+y*) and, for simplicity's sake, we will not be using the Sanskrit terms for the yoga postures. We have also marked where exercises are advanced and where we have offered a more simple variation. Chapter 4 prepares you for exercise by teaching correct breathing, alignment and core strength. Chapter 5 is devoted to the ingredients of a good workout. Read it through before you start, as it will teach you the different moves that can be made with the body. Take your time to learn these fundamental principles.

Then move on to Chapter 6 and start with one exercise from each of the four key sections: a forward bend, backward bend, a rotation and lateral bend. The programme we have built is based on these movements, so experiment, learn the exercises and focus on getting them right. This is also where you begin to exercise intelligently – *you* decide how you want to mix the Pilates and yoga exercises. Vary them each time and see how your body responds. It may be that your body doesn't like a particular movement or finds it difficult. Think about why. If the body is locked or blocked you may need to seek a qualified Pilates or yoga practitioner's help; on the other hand, the exercises may be all you need to release tension. However, if the movements cause you any pain whatsoever, be sure to stop and seek advice.

We have also created four further sections that will help you to become more open in the hips, acquire good shoulder movement, feel the benefits of inverted postures and help you to relax. Only when you are ready attempt the complex, choreographed sequences (from page 187). Then turn to Chapter 7, which gives a variety of balanced workouts using a selection of exercises from each section. By getting to understand the principles you can apply them to the more complex moves and progress in stages, challenging the intelligence of the body further each time you exercise.

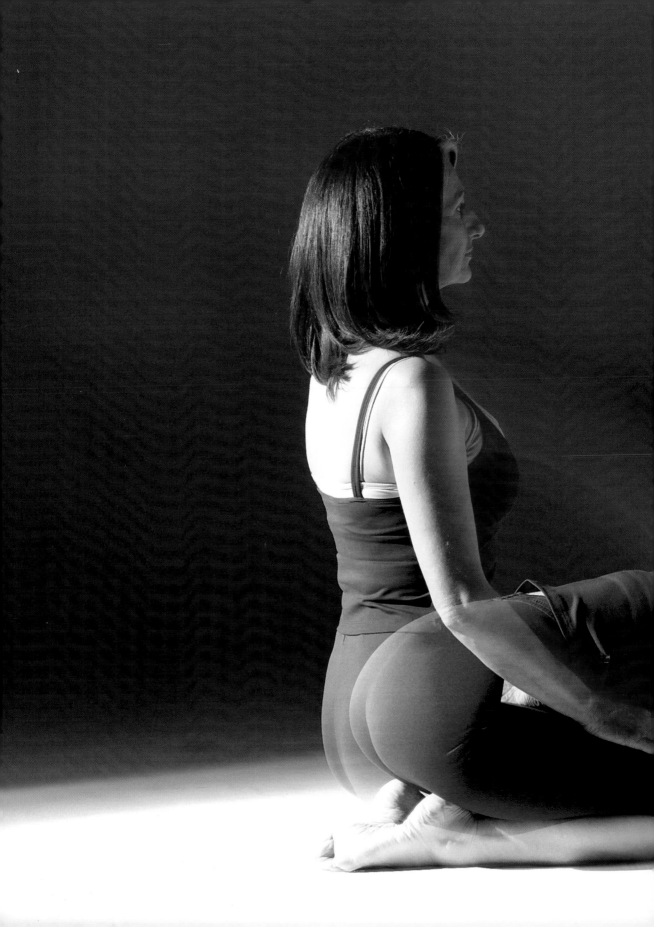

4 Back to basics

Joseph Pilates liked to quote the German philosopher
Schiller, who said: 'It is the mind itself that builds the
body.' In yoga philosophy, there is no separation
between the mind and body. By letting the two work
in harmony, we can create a perfect balance.

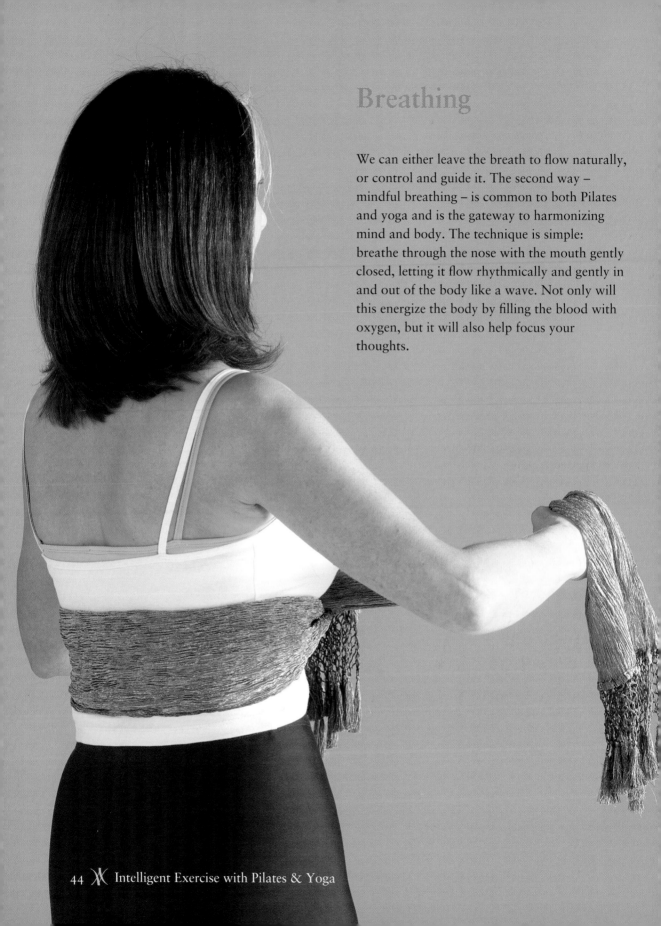

Breathing

We can either leave the breath to flow naturally, or control and guide it. The second way – mindful breathing – is common to both Pilates and yoga and is the gateway to harmonizing mind and body. The technique is simple: breathe through the nose with the mouth gently closed, letting it flow rhythmically and gently in and out of the body like a wave. Not only will this energize the body by filling the blood with oxygen, but it will also help focus your thoughts.

Pilates Breathing

With thoracic or lateral breathing, the lungs become like bellows. The lower ribcage expands wide as you breathe in and closes down as you breathe out. This type of breathing encourages correct movement patterns by enabling you to stay centred while you move.

To practise, try the following:

1 Sit or stand. Wrap a scarf or a towel around your ribs, crossing it over at the front.
2 Holding the opposite ends of the scarf and gently pulling it tight, breathe in and allow your ribs to expand the towel (watch that you do not lift the breastbone too high).
3 As you breathe out, you may squeeze the towel gently to help empty your lungs fully and relax the ribcage, allowing the breast-bone to soften.

Breathing out, you will also engage the pelvic floor and hollow the abdomen (explained in Creating Core Strength on page 54) to give both lumbar and pelvic stability as you move. Ultimately, you will need to keep these abdominal muscles engaged as you breathe in and out.

Yoga Breathing

There are many ways to use the breath in yoga, but all of them use its qualities to energize and connect mind and body. This book deals with a type of breathing generally known as the belly breath.

The other main types of breath commonly used in yoga are: lateral breathing, which is very similar to the breath used here for Pilates, and Ujjayi breath, which is used in forms of yoga like Astanga. Ujjayi breath means victorious breath and is characterized by a gentle purr in the back of the throat.

Belly breathing focuses on the exhalation. In yoga this is known as apana, meaning down breath. This works in harmony with prana, which comes on the in breath. When you use the exhalation fully, the inhalation will come in automatically, filling the lungs without effort. One of the benefits of this breath is found at the end of the exhalation as you wait for the inhalation to move towards you. It is in this stillness that a deep sense of letting go in the body and the mind can be found.

Once connected with the breath, the emphasis is on the fullness, not on the length. The breath can be short, long or a combination of both, but the key is to find a deep breath – one that moves deeply throughout the entire body. Follow the movement that the breath creates (as explained in Yoga Principles page 32) and let the breath guide you without being anxious about it or forcing it.

Most yoga positions are moved into on an exhalation. Once in the position, start connecting with the breath:

- Breathe through the nostrils.
- As you take the exhalation towards its conclusion, focus attention on the abdomen.
- Allow the abdomen to move back towards the spine.
- Notice how the abdomen gently but deeply engages. This is similar to what happens in Pilates when you zip up and hollow.
- Let the breath taper out and wait for the inhalation to move towards you. Allow the body to surrender.
- Let the breath come in freely of its own accord.

Holding Postures

A position should be held for as long as you can breathe fully and evenly, without feeling tension. Your ability will change from day to day, so be content to be in a pose for as long as your body feels able. It takes a minimum of twenty to thirty seconds for a muscle to open out and let go, so don't try to achieve everything in a pose all at once; let it blossom. Don't let tension hold you up in a pose either – come out of it, once it turns from a positive into a negative feeling.

Alignment

This is an area of common ground for Pilates and yoga – we both work with the natural, neutral position of the body. From the head and neck right down through the hips to the feet, the soft, relaxed stance is the same.

For exercise, the body should be in perfect postural alignment. Two good positions for looking at and correcting your alignment are standing and lying down. The Standing Posture is used to find alignment in yoga. In Pilates this Standing Position as well as the Relaxation Position (see page 48) are used to align. We will be referring to both throughout the book as they are often used to start (and in Pilates to finish) exercises, grounding you to the earth and bringing awareness into the body.

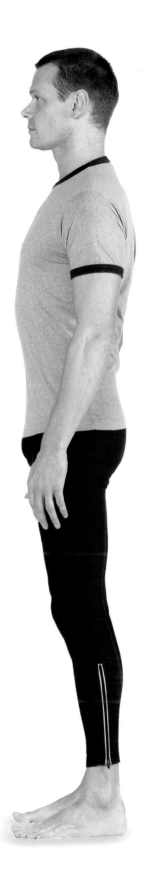

Pilates Alignment

Relaxation Position

1 Lie flat on your back with a small towel or a firm, flat pillow underneath the head, if necessary, to allow the back of the neck to lengthen.

2 Keep your feet parallel and hip-distance apart, your knees bent with your hands placed on the lower abdomen.

3 Release the neck, soften the breastbone and lengthen up through the spine.

4 The pelvis and spine should be in neutral (see the Compass opposite), following their natural tilt and curve, respectively.

5 Your arms are resting lightly on your pelvis – elbows open. (When preparing for exercises have the arms relaxed down by your sides.)

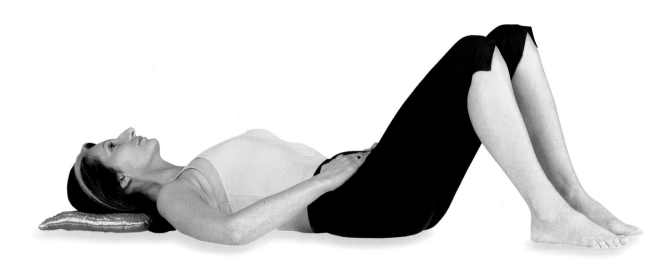

The Compass: Finding Neutral

If you exercise with the pelvis and spine misplaced, you run the risk of creating muscle imbalances and putting the spine under stress. In Pilates, the aim is to have the pelvis and spine in their natural, neutral positions.
To find neutral for these exercises, follow this sequence:

1 Lie in the Relaxation Position (see previous page.)

2 Imagine you have a compass on your lower abdomen. The navel is north and the pubic bone south, with west and east on either side. Now we will do two incorrect positions in order to find the correct one.

3 Tilt your pelvis north. The pelvis will tuck under, the waist will flatten and the curve of the lower back is lost as your tailbone lifts off the floor. You will also grip the muscles around your hips and abdominals.

4 Next, carefully and gently move the pelvis in the other direction so that it tilts south (avoid this bit if you have a back injury). The low back will arch, the ribs will flare and the stomach sticks out. Come back to the starting position.

5 Aim for a neutral position between these two extremes. Go back to the image of the compass and think of the pointer as a spirit level. When you are in neutral, the pubic bone and pelvic bones will be level, and your sacrum will rest squarely on the floor.

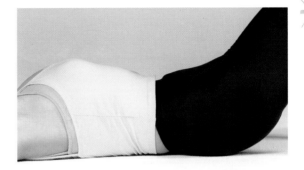

North

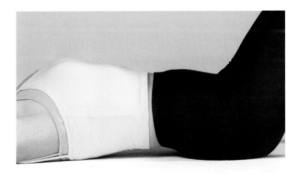

South

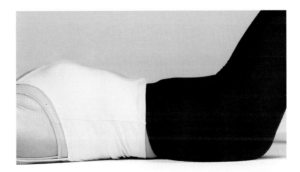

Neutral

Yoga Alignment: Foundation

One of the key aspects of correct alignment in yoga is foundation – the way we connect to the planet. If you built a house without the correct foundation, you wouldn't expect the floor and walls to be straight. The same principle applies to the body (whether standing, sitting or in an inverted posture), so you must begin by giving yourself strong and solid support. To do this, open out your base as much as possible. For each exercise, you will be guided to which part of the body is used as the base, but generally speaking, in a standing posture, your base is the feet; in a sitting posture, the base is the sitting bones; for an inversion (like Downward Facing Dog, see page 180), the base is in the palms of the hands and the balls of the feet; and in a shoulder stand, the base is in the shoulders and the backs of the arms.

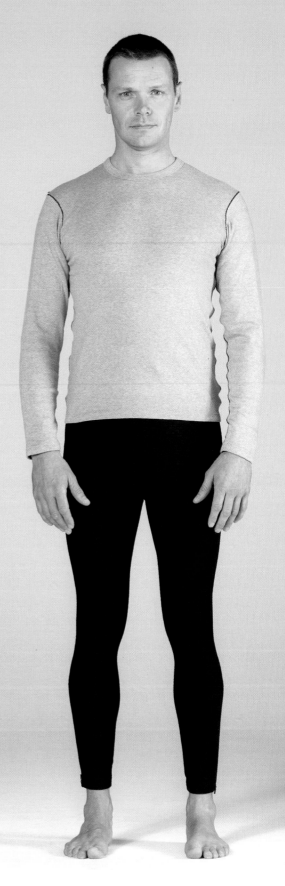

Finding Your Connection

Go back to the image of a house. After laying the foundations properly, the weight must stabilize so that it becomes bedded. Again, it's the same with the body: you have to allow some time for the weight to settle. Then, once grounded, the body is able to discover a security outside itself. This security is the support of the planet. You might already understand that the ground supports us, but intellectual understanding does not automatically translate into an effect on the body. You must feel and be grounded by the force of gravity, not merely understand it. It is then, and only then, that the body can really start to open up.

If you are having difficulty with a position, the first thing to check is your foundation. Without it, you will find that you start to compensate by trying to secure the body in other ways – usually by holding unnecessary tension (in the shoulders or hips for instance), rather than by relying on the core structural muscles.

Once strong foundations are laid, you can start to build. This is perhaps most evident in a standing posture, but it's the same no matter what position you are in.

Standing Posture

No matter what you are doing, the body functions best when it is in proper alignment. In yoga, we find that alignment in the Standing Posture on the following pages. This exercise is often called the Mountain as it has all the majesty that a mountain symbolizes, creating stillness, power and stability. Don't underestimate the importance of this position as it is the basis
of everything you will do: finding your body's alignment now is the best way to understand and improve your yoga practice.

The Feet

1 Start by placing the feet hip-distance apart, parallel to one another.
2 Open out the soles of the feet and stretch your toes. There are twenty-six bones in each foot and getting space between them is the best way to open out the foundation.
3 Distribute the weight evenly between the feet. To do this, transfer the weight gently into the front of the feet and then back into the heels. Finally bring the weight into the middle of the feet, so that the centre of gravity is somewhere over the arch.
4 Keep the arches lifted by keeping the weight central and not letting the feet roll in or out.

The Legs

1 Release the tension in the thighs so the kneecaps drop. You want the legs to relax but not to collapse.
2 The legs should be supportive and straight without locking the back of the knee or extending them towards the wall behind.

The Hips

1 Releasing tension in the thigh will also release the front of the hip.
2 Start to find the relationship between the centre of gravity in the feet and the hips, by feeling that the hips are floating over the feet.
3 Keep this central alignment. If the hips are too far forward, you grip with the front of the hips and the hamstrings. If they are too far back, you grip in the knees and the buttocks.
4 Try and find the fine line where you start to release any superficial tension that you hold unnecessarily.

The Waist

1 When the abdomen moves back towards the spine as you breathe out, the lower back is released and the waist can move out of the hip girdle.
2 Length in the lower back is created when the ribs move away from the hips. Don't impose this movement – let it happen naturally.

The Chest

1 In order for the chest to release so that it can find the centre of gravity over the hips and feet, relax the area between the shoulder blades which usually holds the most tension.
2 Let the shoulder blades move down towards the lower back and soften the breastbone. This allows the front of the chest to open and lift from the inside, and also allows the shoulders to open and release.
3 The chest should float above the hips and feet.

The Head

1 Allow the head to follow the rest of the alignment by gently tucking in the chin so that you are looking towards the horizon. This brings the head back in line and creates length in the back of the neck.
2 Release the superficial tension in the back of the neck and the jaw to let the head float.

Levity

Most of us do one of two things when standing: we either collapse, which results in bad posture, or we do the opposite and push away from the planet. The latter is usually seen when someone is trying to stretch and lengthen – tight knees, chest and shoulders pulled up, spine pushed forward, perhaps with the hands above the head and the fingertips stretched towards the ceiling, closing down the back of the neck and locking off the elbows. This may seem better than a slouch and may even feel good, but when you extend in this way, you do nothing but create tension.

Both of these extremes fail to make use of the natural ability of the body to support itself through its skeletal structure and stabilizing core. What you will find if you stand in open, correct alignment and yield towards the planet is that gravity can pull and lift you at the same time. Standing becomes effortless: as you release superficial tension in the body, there is a strong sense of grounding but also of lightness. As the weight goes down with the gravitational pull, an amazing thing happens, like a bouncing ball, you receive something back called levity. This levity is the rebounding gravitational force that lifts and opens you out from your centre and you become like a tree: rooted from the waist down and growing from the waist up. This feeling of levity cannot be imposed, but can only come about once we develop a free and mobile core.

Creating Core Strength

Some exercises concentrate on internal
movement – you may not feel that you are
doing very much, but the precision and control
gained from these subtle changes in the body
play an essential part in building strength from
the core outwards. How you control these
muscles during exercise is usually thought of
as an area of conflict between Pilates and yoga,
but in fact we found that they use the same
principles once the obstacle of different
terminology is removed.

Pilates Core Strength

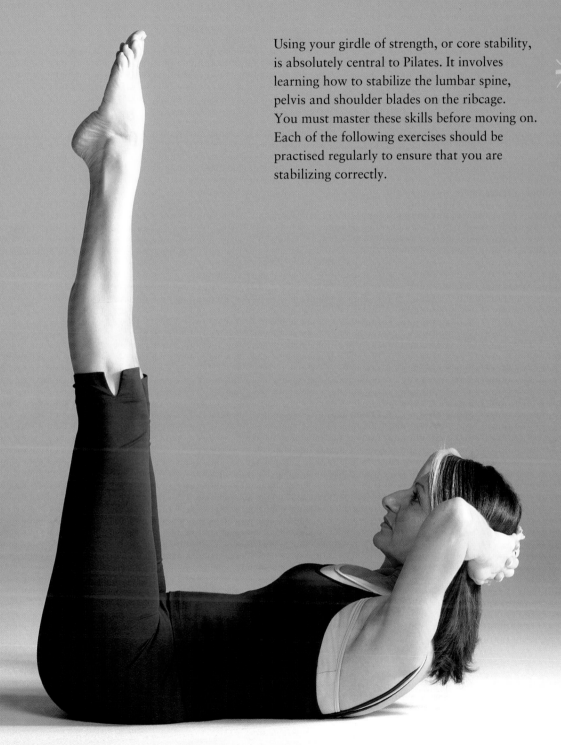

Using your girdle of strength, or core stability, is absolutely central to Pilates. It involves learning how to stabilize the lumbar spine, pelvis and shoulder blades on the ribcage. You must master these skills before moving on. Each of the following exercises should be practised regularly to ensure that you are stabilizing correctly.

The Pelvic Elevator (Sitting)

Aim

This exercise was created to isolate and engage the deep stabilizing muscles of the pelvis, pelvic floor and spine – transversus abdominis and multifidus. In order to achieve the best possible stability, you need to be able to contract the pelvic floor muscles at the same time as hollowing the lower abdominals to engage tranversus abdominis.

Initially, it is not easy to isolate and engage the pelvic floor muscles and takes considerable concentration. The pelvic floor is the muscles of the vagina for women and the urethra for both sexes (men should think about lifting their 'crown jewels'!). One way to help locate these muscles is to suck your thumb as you draw them up inside. It sounds crazy, but it works! At this stage we do not want you to engage the muscles around the anus, as it is too easy for the buttock muscles to kick in and substitute. If possible, try to draw the pelvic floor together from side to side, like the shutter of a camera lens closing, this helps good recruitment.

Once you have found the pelvic floor muscles, it should be easier to isolate the tranversus abdominis. To engage these muscles correctly (at no more than 20 per cent) think of:

- hollowing
- scooping
- drawing back the abdominals towards the spine
- sucking in

Preparation

Sit on an upright chair making sure that you are sitting square, with your weight even on both buttocks. Imagine that your pelvic floor is like the lift in a building and this exercise requires you to take the lift up to different floors of the building.

Action

1 Breathe in wide and full into your back and sides, then lengthen up through the spine.
2 As you breathe out, draw up the muscles of the pelvic floor as if you are trying to prevent the flow of urine (see notes above). Take the pelvic lift up to the first floor of the building. Notice your lower abdominals hollow.
3 Breathe in and release the lift back to the ground floor.
4 Breathe out and now take the lift up to the second floor.
5 Breathe in and release.
6 Breathe out and take the lift up to the third/fourth floor. Notice how when you do this, the superficial upper abdominals automatically engage.
7 Breathe in and relax.

Watchpoints

- When you reached the first floor, you should have felt the deep lower abdominals engage. This is transversus abdominis coming into play. By starting the action from underneath, you encourage the 'six pack' muscle, rectus abdominis, to stay quiet. If you were to take the lift all the way to the top floor, the third floor or above, you would probably be engaging the muscles at over 30 per cent and the rectus abdominis would take over – so keep the action low and gentle.
- Do not allow the buttock muscles to join in.
- Keep your jaw relaxed.
- Don't take your shoulders up to the top floor as well – keep them down and relaxed.
- Try not to grip around your hips.
- Keep the pelvis and spine quite still.

Once you have found your pelvic floor muscles, learn how to engage them in different positions.

The following three positions will help to ensure that this is done correctly:

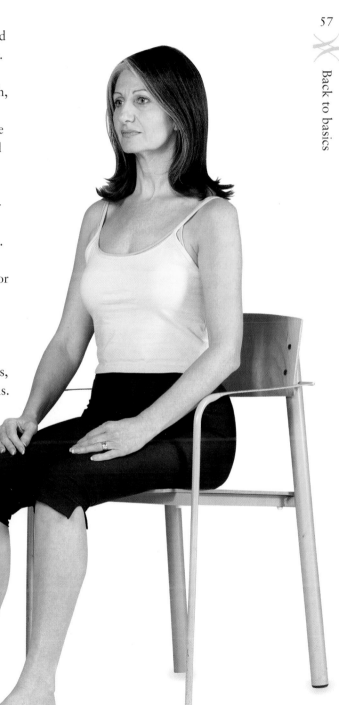

Stabilizing on All Fours

Try this wearing only your underwear with a mirror underneath you. This way, you can check to see if your six pack muscle remains quiet. Allow your abdominals to relax.

Preparation
- Kneel on all fours with your hands beneath your shoulders and your knees beneath your hips.
- Have the top of your head lengthening away from your tailbone and your pelvis in neutral. It helps to imagine that there is a small pool of water resting at the base of your spine.

Action
1 Breathe in to prepare.
2 Breathe out and zip up and hollow. Your back should not move.
3 Breathe in and release.
4 Now try to keep zipped while breathing in and out.

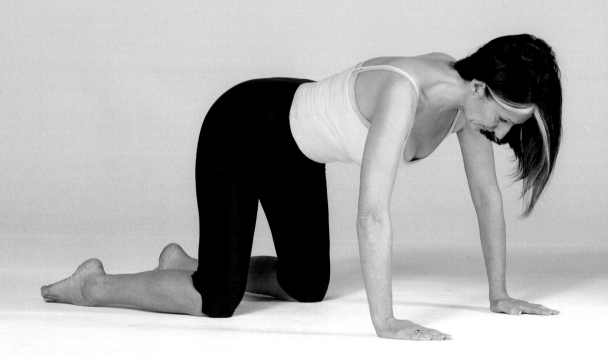

Stabilizing in Prone Lying

Preparation

- Lie face down, resting your head on your folded hands.
- Open the shoulders out and relax the upper back (use a small, flat cushion under your abdomen if your lower back is uncomfortable).
- Your legs are relaxed and your feet are shoulder-distance apart.

Action

1 Breathe in to prepare.
2 Breathe out, zip up from the pelvic floor and draw the lower abdominals away from the floor.
3 Try imagining that there is a precious egg on the floor just above the pubic bone that must not be crushed. Do not tighten the buttocks. There should be no movement in the pelvis or the spine.
4 Breathe in and release.
5 Once again, try to stay zipped as you breath in and out.

This then, is your strong centre. For most of the exercises, you will be asked to zip up and hollow, engaging the pelvic floor muscles and drawing the lower abdominals back to the spine, before and during your movements, and lengthening away from a strong centre. Remember always keep the action low and gentle. **But note that for the Advanced exercises when both legs are raised from the floor you will be working the deep abdominal much harder to keep your back anchored.**

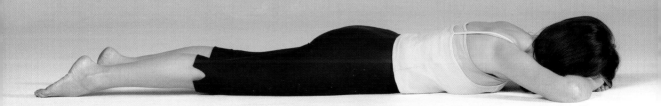

Stabilizing in the Relaxation Position

Preparation

Lie in the Relaxation Position (see page 48). Check that your pelvis is in neutral.

Action

1 Breathe in to prepare and lengthen through the top of your head.
2 Breathe out, zip up and hollow – your abdominals almost sink back towards the spine.
3 Do not allow the pelvis to tuck under. Do not push into the spine. Keep your tailbone on the floor and lengthening away.
4 Breathe in and relax.

When you can do this easily, practise zipping up and hollowing on both the in and out breath. Use lateral thoracic breathing, wide and full into your sides and back, staying zipped.

You must be careful not to tuck the pelvis under (tilting north). If you do, you will lose your neutral position. It also means that other muscles – the rectus abdominis and the hip flexors – are doing the work instead of the transversus abdominis and the internal obliques. Put your hand under your waist to check if you are pushing into the spine. Once you have learned to create a strong centre, you can add movements such as rotation, flexion and extension.

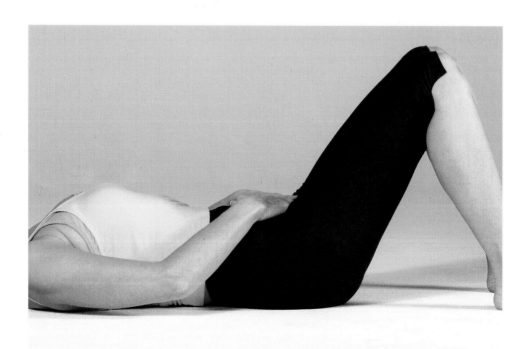

Pelvic Stability
(Leg Slides, Drops, Folds and Turn Out)

Aim

Having mastered breathing, correct alignment and the creation of a strong centre, you can now learn how to add movement co-ordinating all this. It isn't easy to begin with, but it soon becomes automatic. Meanwhile, the process of learning this co-ordination is fabulous mental and physical training as it stimulates that two-way communication between the brain and the muscles.

Start with small movements then build up to more complicated combinations. Below are four movements to practise, all of them requiring you to keep the pelvis completely still. A useful image to have is that you have a set of car headlamps on your pelvis, shining at the ceiling. The beam should be fixed, rather than mimicking searchlights! You can vary which exercises you practise each session but the preparation position is the same for all four.

Preparation

- Adopt the Relaxation Position (see page 48).
- Check that your pelvis is in neutral, tailbone down and lengthening away, then place your hands on your pelvic bones to check for unwanted movement.

Action for Leg Slides

1 Breathe in wide and full to prepare.
2 Breathe out and zip up and hollow.
3 Slide one leg away along the floor in line with your hips and keep the lower abdominals engaged and the pelvis still, stable and in neutral.
4 Breathe into your lower ribcage while you return the leg to the bent position, trying to keep the stomach hollow. If you cannot yet breathe in and maintain a strong centre, take an extra breath and return the leg on the out breath.
5 Repeat five times with each leg.

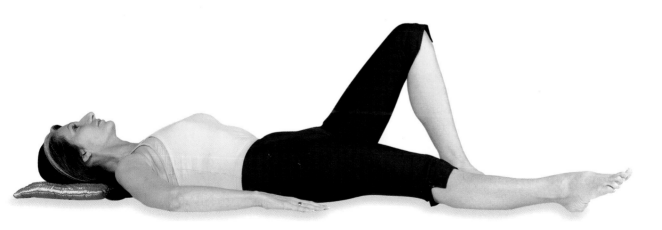

Action for Knee Drops

1 Breathe in wide and full to prepare.
2 Breathe out, zip up and hollow, and allow one knee to open slowly to the side. Go only as far as the pelvis can stay still.
3 Breathe in, still zipped and hollowed, as the knee returns to centre.
4 Repeat five times with each leg.

Action for Knee Folds

With this movement it is particularly useful to feel that the muscles stay 'scooped' and do not bulge while you fold the knee in. Very gently feel the muscles engage as you zip up and hollow.

1 Breathe in wide and full to prepare.
2 Breathe out, zip up and hollow, then fold the left knee up. Think of the thighbone dropping down into the hip and anchoring there.
3 Do not lose your neutral pelvis – the tailbone stays down – and do not rely on the other leg to stabilize you. Imagine your foot is on a cream cake and you don't want to press down on it.
4 Breathe in and hold.
5 Breathe out still zipped and hollowed as you slowly return the foot to the floor.
6 Repeat five times with each leg

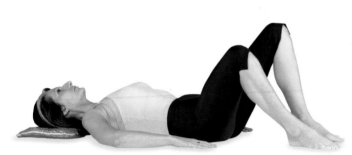

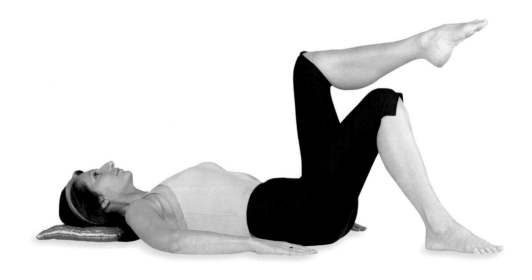

Action for Turning Out the Leg

This next action involves turning the leg out from the hip and is a preparation for exercises where the legs are held in a turned-out position. It works the deep gluteal muscles, especially gluteus medius, which is one of the main stabilizing muscles of the pelvis.

Warning: please take advice if you suffer from sciatica.

1 Breathe in wide and full to prepare.
2 Breathe out, zip up and hollow, then fold the right knee up. Think of the thighbone dropping down into the hip and anchoring there.
3 Breathe in then out, zip up and hollow and turn the right leg out from the hip bringing the right foot to touch the left knee if you can.
4 Do not allow the pelvis to tilt or twist or turn, keep it central and stable. (Remember the headlamps glued to the ceiling!)
5 Breathe in and then out and zip up and hollow as you reverse the movement to return the foot to the floor.
6 Repeat five times to each side.

Watchpoints

- Remember that you are trying to avoid even the slightest movement of the pelvis. It helps to think of the waist being long and even on both sides as you make the movement.
- Try to keep your neck and jaw released throughout.

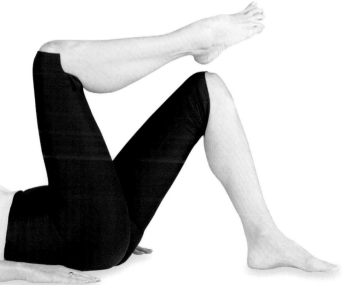

Scapular Stability

The final part of our girdle of strength involves learning how to stabilize the shoulder blades and move the upper body correctly with good mechanics. For this, you need to find the muscles lower trapezius and serratus anterior that set the shoulder blades down into the back, holding them in just the right position to allow the arm to move freely and easily and the shoulder joint to be correctly positioned.

To find these muscles, try the exercise opposite.

Back view   **Side view**

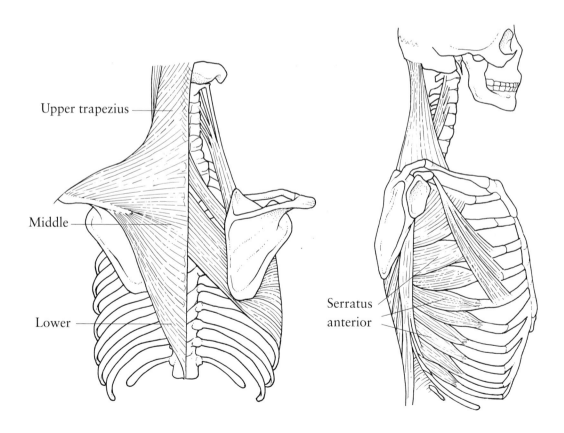

Upper trapezius

Middle

Lower

Serratus anterior

The Dart (Stage One)

Equipment
A flat pillow (optional).

Preparation
- Lie face down (you can place a flat pillow under your forehead to allow you to breathe) with your arms by your sides and your palms facing up.
- Your neck is long, legs relaxed but in parallel.

Action
1 Breathe in to prepare and lengthen through the spine, tucking your chin in gently as if you were holding a ripe peach beneath it.
2 Breathe out, zip up and hollow, and slide your shoulder blades down into your back, lifting your head slightly, lengthening your fingers down towards your feet and turning the hands to face the body.
3 The top of your head stays lengthening away from you.

4 Keep looking straight down at the floor. Do not tip your head back.
5 Breathe in and feel the length of the body from the tips of your toes to the top of your head.
6 Breathe out, still zipping, and release.

Watchpoints
- Keep hollowing the lower abdominals.
- Do not strain the neck – it should feel released as your shoulders engage down into your back. Think of a swan's neck growing out between its wings.
- Keep your feet on the floor.
- Stop if you feel at all uncomfortable in the low back.

This exercise can also be done with the feet hip-width apart and the thigh and buttock muscles relaxed.

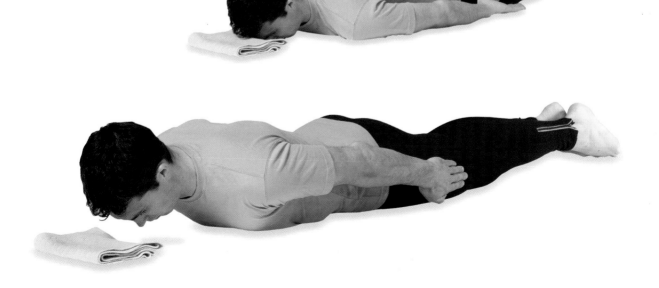

Moving On . . .

The muscles you felt drawing your shoulder blades down into your back are the stabilizing muscles – lower trapezius and serratus anterior. Now that you have located them, try to feel them working in this next exercise.

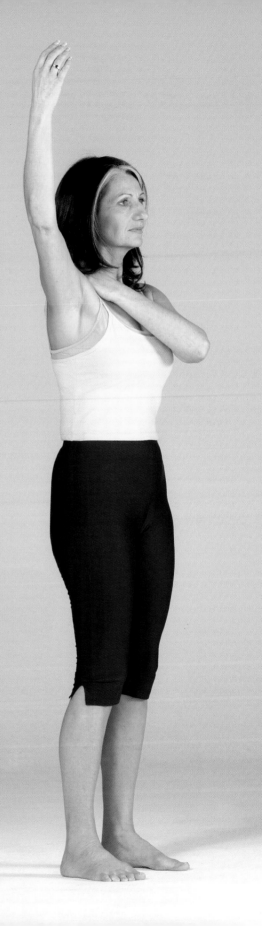

Floating Arms

Aim
To learn correct upper-body mechanics.

Preparation
- Begin in the Standing Posture (page 51).
- Place your left hand on your right shoulder to check that the upper part of your trapezius muscle remains 'quiet' for as long as possible. Very often this will overwork as the arm rises, so think of it staying soft and released.

Action

1. Breathe in to prepare and lengthen up through the spine, letting the neck relax.
2. Breathe out and zip up and hollow. Slowly begin to raise the right arm, reaching wide out of the shoulder blades like a bird's wing. Think of the hand as leading the arm; the arm following the hand as it floats upwards.
3. Rotate the arm so that when it reaches shoulder level the palm is open to the ceiling. Try to keep the shoulder under your hand as still as possible and the shoulder blades dropping down into your back as long as possible.
4. Breathe in as you lower the arms to your side.
5. Repeat three times with each arm.

Watchpoints
- Keep a sense of openness in the upper body.
- Do not allow your upper body to shift to the side, keep centred.
- As the arm floats up, think of the shoulder blade sliding down to begin with and then coiling outwards on the ribcage.

The Starfish

Aim

To combine everything you have learnt so far!

Stage One: The Upper Body

Preparation

• Lie in the Relaxation Position (see page 48).

Action

1 Breathe wide into your lower ribcage to prepare.
2 Breathe out, zip up and hollow, and start to take one arm back in a backstroke movement as if to touch the floor behind your head. You may not be able to touch the floor comfortably so only move the arm as far as is comfortable.

3 Do not force it – keep it soft and open with the elbow bent. Think of the shoulder blade connecting down into your back. The ribs are down and stay calm. Do not allow the back to arch at all.
4 Breathe in as you return the arm to your side.
5 Repeat five times with each arm.

Watchpoint

• Not everyone can touch the floor behind them without arching the upper back, so do not strain. It is better to keep the back down than force the arm.

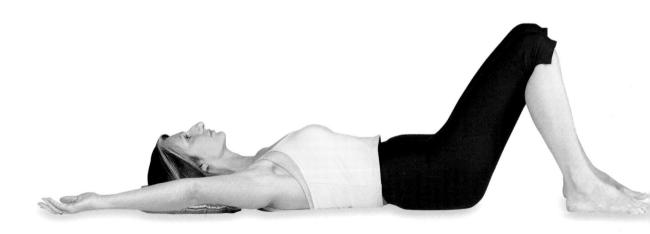

Stage Two: The Full Starfish

Now we are going to co-ordinate the opposite arm and leg movement away from our strong centre. Although this looks simple, it is a sophisticated movement pattern, using all the skills of good movement learnt so far.

Preparation
- Lie in the Relaxation Position (see page 48).

Action
1 Breathe in wide and full to prepare.
2 Breathe out, zip up and hollow. Slide the left leg away along the floor in a line with your hips and take the right arm above you in a backstroke movement.
3 Keep the pelvis completely neutral, stable and still, and the stomach muscles engaged.

4 Keep a sense of width and openness in the upper body and shoulders, and think of the shoulder blades sliding down into your back.
5 Breathe in, still zipped and hollowed, and return the limbs to the Relaxation Position.
6 Repeat five times alternating arms and legs.

Watchpoints
- Do not be tempted to overreach – the girdle of strength must stay in place – yet keep the actions flowing and natural.
- Slide the leg in a line with the hip.

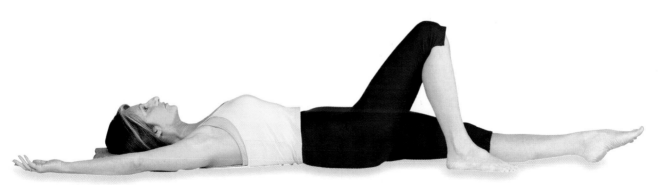

Neck Rolls and Chin Tucks

Aim

This exercise will release tension from the neck, freeing the cervical spine. It also uses the deep stabilizers of the neck, the anterior sub-occipitals, and lengthens the neck extensors.

Another important aspect in re-educating the head–neck relationship lies in the relative strength of the neck extensors (which tilt the head back) and flexors (which tilt the head forward). If you think about the body positioned at a desk or at a steering wheel, the head is usually thrust forward and tipped back, causing a muscle imbalance. The superficial neck flexors need to be released and the deep neck flexors engaged. By relaxing the jaw, lengthening the back of the neck and gently tucking in the chin, this balance can be redressed.

Please take note that this is a subtle movement – you should tuck your chin in gently.

Equipment

A flat pillow (optional).

Preparation

- Lie in the Relaxation Position (see page 48) with your arms resting on your lower abdomen.
- Only use a flat pillow for this if you are uncomfortable without one (your head will roll better if you do not use one).

Action

1 Release your neck and jaw, allowing your tongue to widen at its base. Keep the neck nicely lengthened and soften your breastbone. Allow the shoulder blades to widen and melt into the floor.
2 Now, allow your head to roll slowly to one side.
3 Bring it back to the centre and over to the other side, taking your time.
4 When the neck feels free, bring the head to the centre and gently tuck in your chin, as if holding a ripe peach under it. Keep the head on the floor and lengthen out of the back of the neck.
5 Return the head to the centre.
6 Repeat the rolling to the side and chin tuck eight times.

Watchpoints

• Do not force the head or neck – just let it roll naturally.
• Do not lift the head off the floor when you tuck the chin in.

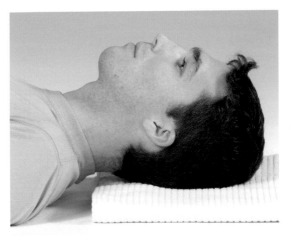

Neutral

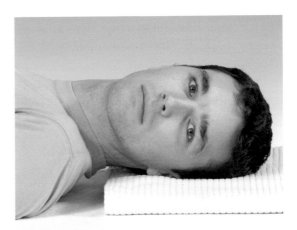

Release to one side

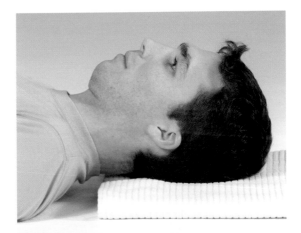

Chin tucks

Yoga Core Strength

Core strength is one of the keys to the practice of yoga and is referred to as the bandhas which means to bond or to lock and is the equivalent to stabilizing in Pilates. There are three such locks:

- Mula-bandha (root lock) is the same as engaging the pelvic floor.
- Uddiyana-bandha (upward lock) is the same as stabilizing the abdomen by hollowing it back towards the spine. This works in the same way as zipping up and hollowing does in Pilates.
- In jalandhar-bandha (throat lock) the chin is tucked in so you are looking towards the horizon. This lengthens the back of the neck and stabilizes the chest and shoulders.

All of these bandhas start to come naturally with correct alignment. But as they need to work for long periods of time, do not exert too much pressure on them – it is sufficient to have them subtly engaged, as explained in The Principles of the Body (see page 18).

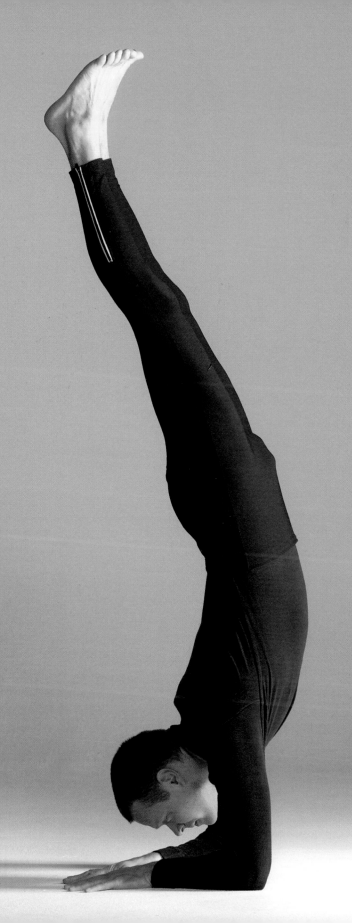

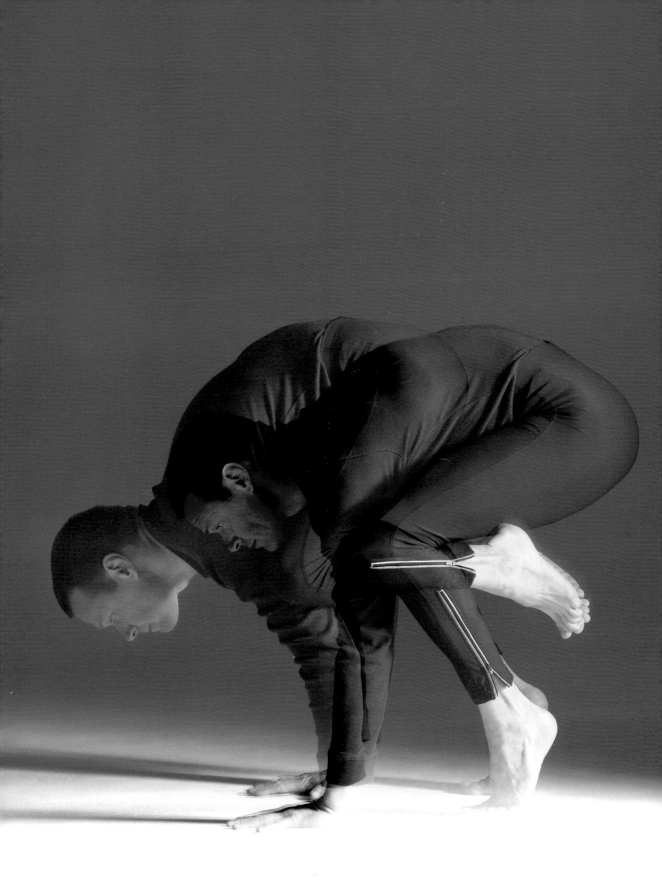

5 The ingredients of a good workout

There is good movement and bad movement, and therefore good exercise and bad exercise. So what made us choose these exercises and think that they would complement each other? Put simply, you only have one body and it can only move in certain ways. There are four main movements that the trunk of the body is capable of doing using the spine – flexion, extension, rotation and lateral flexion. The body can move normally using a combination of these. For each movement, we have chosen a selection of exercises from both Pilates and yoga, and by concentrating on these groups first you will begin to understand how the body moves. Sometimes the basis of your exercise will be on flexibility, sometimes it will be on strength, but each exercise will work with the spine. Then, to balance your workout and make it more varied and dynamic we have added exercises to promote good alignment and movement for the pelvis and hips and the shoulders. The final sections focus on inversely flowing sequences and relaxation.

In Chapter 7, we have put together a choice of workouts using a selection of exercises for each movement and incorporating balancing and strengthening exercises for flexibility. Some will be invigorating and energizing, others will be relaxing and calming, but each allows you to work intelligently by choosing how you want to exercise.

Understanding the Spine

In the womb, the spine grows to its natural shape, but the more pronounced curves of the spine develop during early childhood enabling it to absorb some of the shock that would otherwise be transmitted to the head when the body moves. When the body is standing, the postural muscles work constantly to keep it upright. There exists a delicate balance between those muscles at the front of the body and those at the back – any habitual change in the way the body stands or sits will affect that balance.

The spinal ligaments are affected in a similar way. If you repeatedly bend forwards or backwards, the balance is upset. Furthermore, the pressure within the spinal discs will increase. Sitting slumped over a desk all day alters the angles of the curves of the spine and stresses the ligaments, muscles and discs. Eventually, pain can set in. This is why these exercises are done with the spine in a neutral position, maintaining its length and natural curves to avoid compression.

In a healthy back, all the segments of the spine work together to create the desired movement. Each vertebra contributes to that movement – a bit like a bicycle chain. However if one level becomes locked, by poor posture for example, the chain is upset and areas of the back become jammed. Often the levels above and below the locked area become over-flexible to compensate, making the back hypo-mobile (not enough movement) in one area and hyper-mobile (too much movement) above and/or below. This puts an enormous strain on the back.

The importance of both the spine and its health is common to both Pilates and yoga.

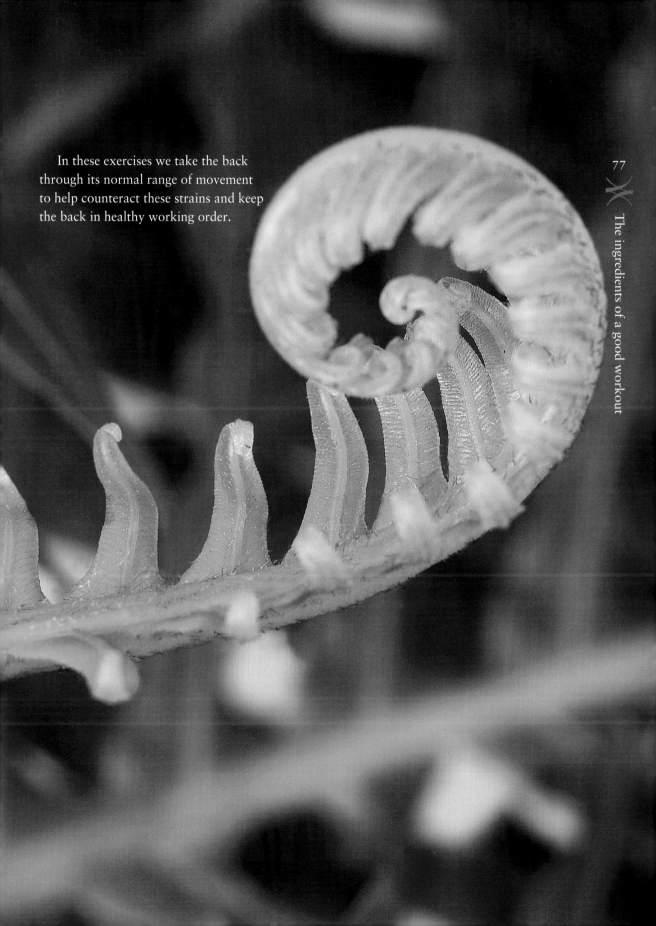

In these exercises we take the back through its normal range of movement to help counteract these strains and keep the back in healthy working order.

The Pelvis and Hips

Two thirds of the world's population have no difficulty in squatting, whether to rest, sit or eat, yet it is unusual to see anyone in that position in the West. The explanation is simple: chairs. Put into chairs from around six months old, Westerners often find that their hips are not as open as that of their Eastern counterparts and so need to work on increasing flexibility in this area. You need a similar amount of movement potential in the hips as you have in the spine. They need to be capable of flexion, extension, adduction and abduction, external and internal rotation. By moving the hips in these ways you lubricate the joints, ensuring correct alignment and preventing daily wear and tear, all of which contribute to their health and mobility. We will help create openness in the hips by taking you through this range of movements in your workout.

The pelvis is connected to the spine. It is balanced on the hip joints and can tilt one way or the other, pulling the lumbar spine with it, which stresses the spinal tissues. Learning to find your neutral pelvic position and achieving pelvic stability will help to balance the whole body.

The Shoulders

Modern life – from using computers to couch-potato sitting – closes the body down. Not only does the spine round forward, but the shoulders rotate and tension tightens the muscles. Add to this the way in which the head is poked forward and you have the muscles of the shoulders and neck – the upper trapezius, levator scapulae, anterior deltoids, the pectorals and the superficial neck muscles, in particular the sternocleidomastoid – all shortened and over-working. While these muscles grow increasingly tense, the muscles of the mid-back, especially lower trapezius and serratus anterior, are held overstretched and lengthened and the deep neck flexors, the sub-occipital muscles, are weak – the shoulder blades themselves may even be held in a winged position. The shoulder exercises in this book create flexibility in the upper body, opening out the chest and strengthening the muscles which stabilize the shoulder blades to encourage correct alignment and good shoulder mechanics.

Inversion

More common in yoga, inverted postures are thought to be of great benefit to your internal organs as well as to the cardiovascular, lymphatic and nervous systems. Research suggests that inverted postures relieve pressure on the heart and arteries, encouraging venous return to benefit the circulation of blood around the body. This process also stimulates the lymph system, responsible for eliminating toxins and waste. Inverting is thought to be particularly good for those with high stress levels, but should be avoided during menstruation (the veins in the uterus are fragile and should not be congested with blood).

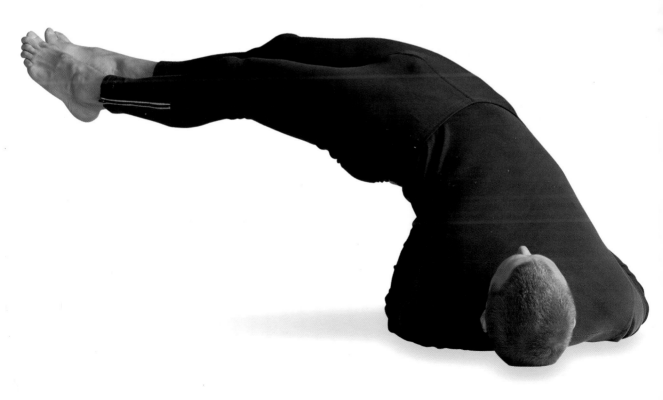

Flowing Sequences

As you work your way through Chapter 6
you will gain the skills you need to perform
the complex, choreographed sequences which
comprise the last section in the chapter before
relaxation. This book is all about movement
and moving well, so once you have gone
through all the motions that the body is capable
of and learned to do them properly, put them
together into these sequences to bring complete
balance to each workout.

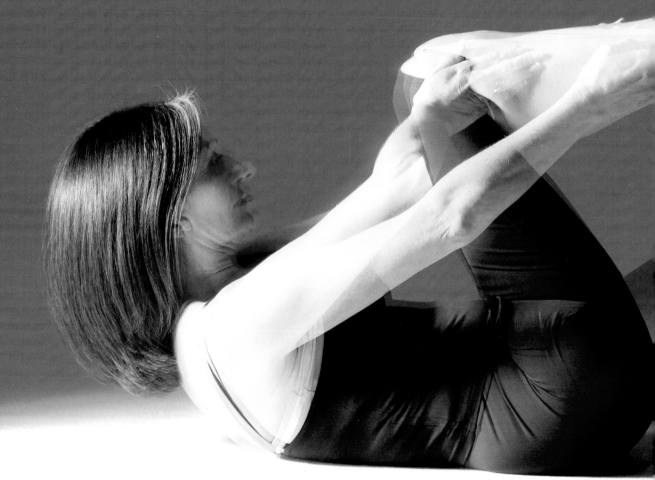

Relaxation

Some of the exercises in this book are very
stimulating, but it's also important to relax.
Both Pilates and yoga work with the release of
over-dominant muscles that hold tension in the
body – tension that is often so deep that even
when it is released, the body picks it up again at
the slightest movement. The relaxation exercises
will help you relax muscles effectively and over
a sustained period so that when you do finish
your programme, you should continue to feel
the benefits.

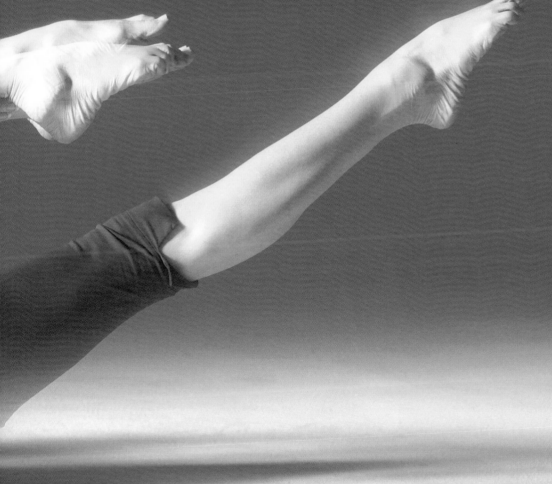

And Finally . . .

This programme is designed to give you a range
of simple movements suitable for doing at
home. We have not included any weight,
aerobic or resistance work, which you should
try to do at other times for a balanced body
as well as for bone and cardiovascular health.

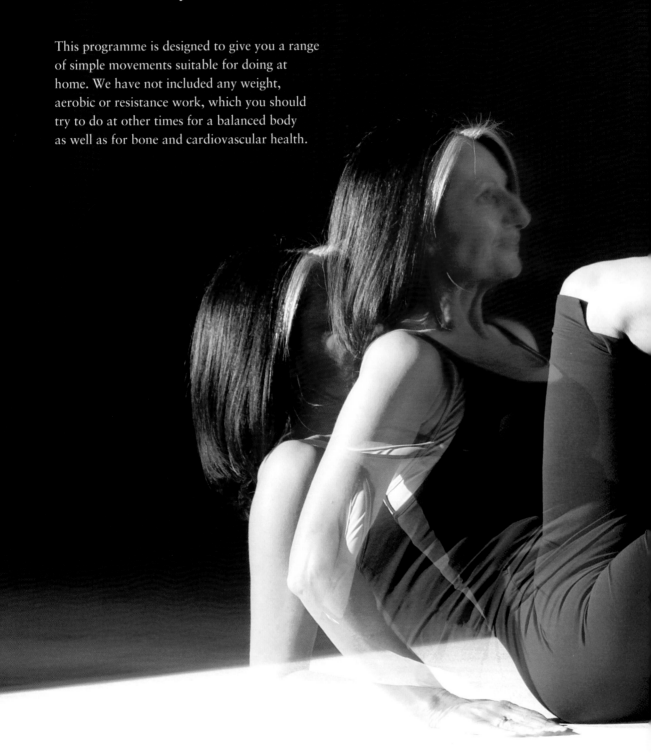

6 The programme

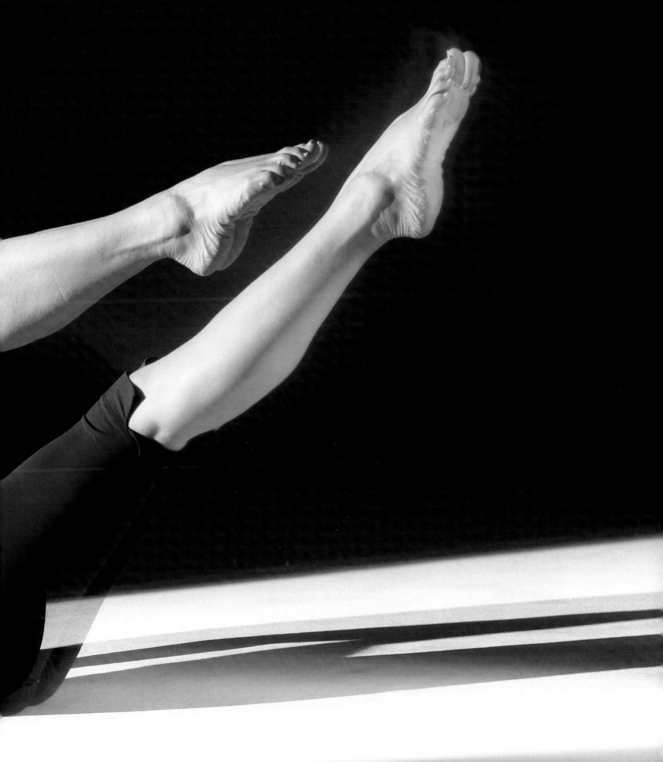

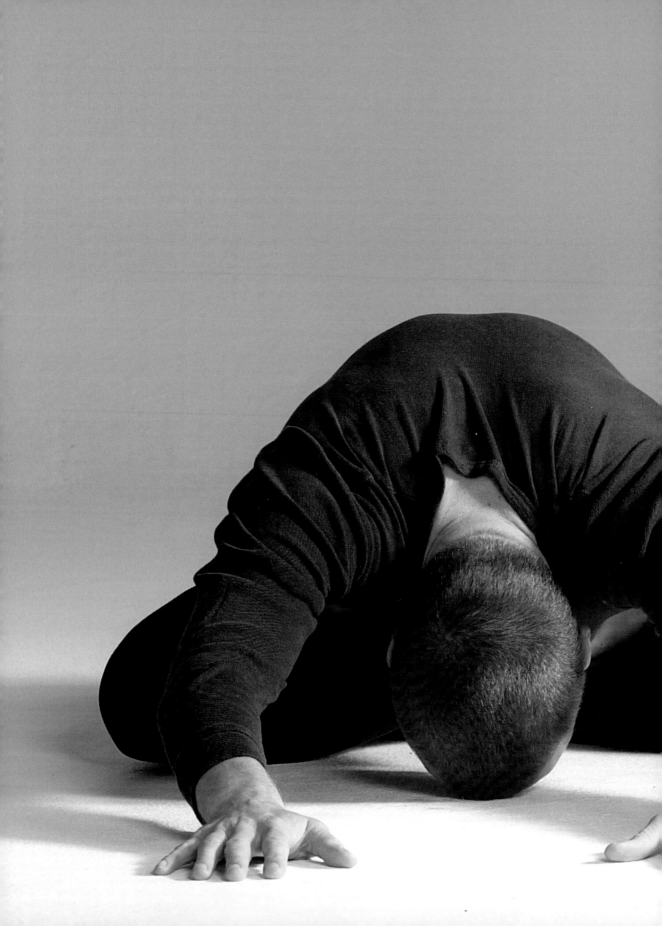

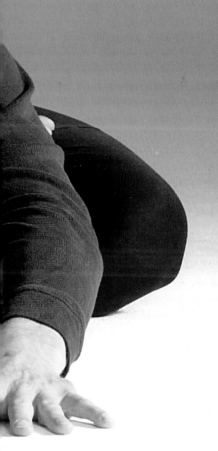

Flexion/
Forward Bend

Beach Ball Hamstring Stretch (p)

Aim

This exercise opens the joints in the spine as well as stretching out the hamstring muscles, which are often tight when the body is out of alignment. It also reinforces scapular stability and deep breathing.

Warning: take advice if you have a knee or hip problem.

Preparation

- Sit squarely on the floor with your knees bent and the soles of your feet together. You should be comfortable.
- Straighten the left leg out in front of you, parallel to the hip and with the kneecap facing straight up. The sole of your right foot moves to rest on the inside of the left calf or knee. (If this becomes uncomfortable, try sitting on a rolled up towel.) Do not lock the knees.
- Check that this action doesn't twist the pelvis and that you are sitting on your sitting bones.

Action

1 Breathe in wide and full to prepare and lengthen the space between the hips and the ribcage. As you breathe out, zip up and hollow, lift up from your hips and gently curl the spine stretching forward as if coming up and over a large beach ball.

2 Stay centred and keep the weight even on your sitting bones.

3 Keep your neck long, your chin gently tucked in, sliding the shoulder blades down towards the waist. Keep the arm alongside the straight leg relaxed and rest the other hand behind you with the palm facing upwards.

4 Follow the breath for five breaths. On the next breath out, zip up and hollow before gently rebuilding the spine, vertebra by vertebra, until you are sitting upright. Repeat on the other side.

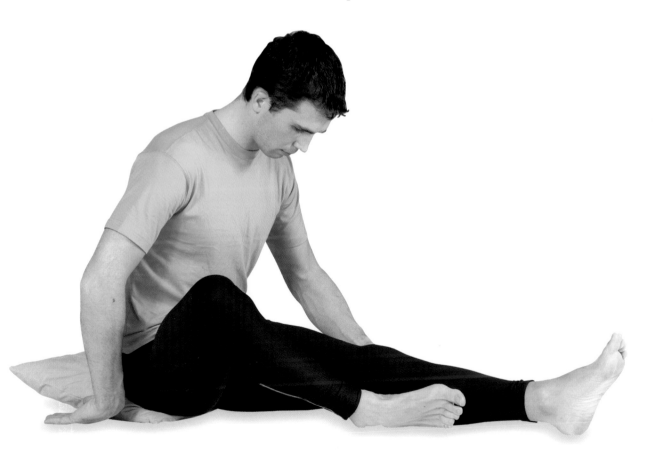

Curl Up (*p*)

Aim
With perfect postural alignment, this exercise will strengthen the abdominals for a flatter stomach, when the muscles are engaged in the correct order.

Warning: avoid this exercise if you have neck problems or osteoporosis of the spine.

Preparation
• Lie in the Relaxation Position (see page 48) and gently release the neck by slowly rolling the head from side to side.

Action
1 Lightly clasp both hands behind your head, allowing them to cradle and support the head without pulling the neck. Tuck in the chin as if you are holding a delicate ripe peach under it.
2 Breathe in wide and full to prepare. As you breathe out, zip up and hollow (stay zipped throughout).
3 Soften the breastbone, and curl up.
4 Keep the length and width in the front of the pelvis, with the tailbone down on the floor lengthening away from the ribcage. Do not allow the lower abdominals to bulge – they must stay hollowed.
5 Breathe in and slowly curl back down.
6 Repeat up to ten times.

Watchpoints
• Try not to grip around the hips.
• Stay in neutral, tailbone down on the floor and lengthening away. The front of the body keeps its length – a useful image is that there is a strip of sticky tape along the front of the body that should not wrinkle.

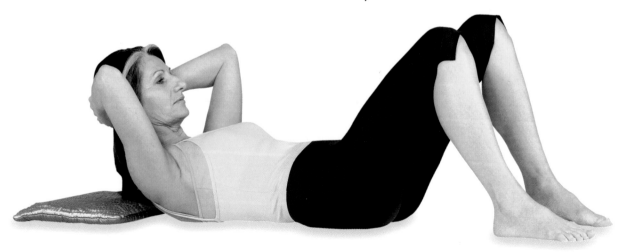

Oblique Curl Up (p)

Aim
This exercise works the oblique muscles.

Warning: avoid this exercise if you have neck problems.

Preparation
- Lie in the Relaxation Position (see page 48) and place both hands behind your head, keeping the elbows open and just forward of your ears. Tuck the chin in gently.

Action
1 Breathe in wide and full to prepare.
2 Breathe out, zip up and hollow, and bring your left shoulder across towards your right knee. The elbow stays back – it is the shoulder that moves forward.
3 Your stomach must stay hollow, with the pelvis stable.
4 Breathe in and lower.
5 Repeat five times to each side.

Watchpoints
- Make sure that the pelvis stays square and stable.
- Keep the upper body open.
- Keep the neck released.

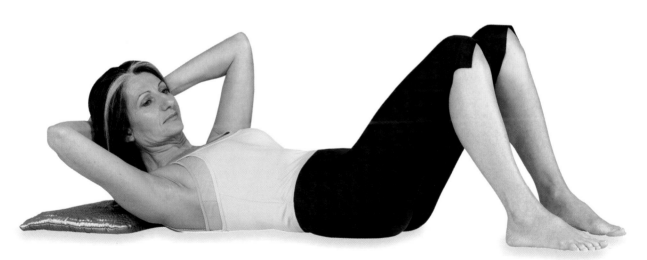

The Hundred (p)

Aim
The Hundred is a classical Pilates exercise and was traditionally the warm-up for mat classes. It has been broken down into manageable sections here so that you take time to master the breathing pattern that stimulates the circulatory system before proceeding. This exercise strengthens the pectoral muscles and abdominals, while helping you master stabilizing the shoulder blades.

Equipment for all stages
A firm, flat cushion (optional).

Stage One: Breathing

1 Lie in the Relaxation Position (see page 48), with your head on the cushion if it is more comfortable, and place your hands on your lower ribcage.
2 Breathe in wide and full, into your sides and back, for a count of five.
3 Breathe out and zip up and hollow, for a count of five.
4 Repeat ten times, trying to stay zipped and hollowed for both the in and the out breaths. If you find the count of five too difficult, try the count of three.

Stage Two: Arm Action

Preparation
- Lie in the Relaxation Position (see page 48), with the cushion under your head if it is more comfortable.
- Your arms are a few centimetres off the floor. The palms should be facing down, fingers long.
- Keep the shoulders down and a sense of openness in the upper body.

Action
1 Breathe in wide and full to prepare.
2 Pump the arms up and down for a count of five, no more than 15 centimetres from the floor. Reach through the fingertips.
3 Breathe out and pump the arms up and down for a count of five.
4 Repeat up to ten times.

Stage Three

Preparation
- Lie in the Relaxation Position (see page 48), with your head on the cushion if it is more comfortable.
- Zip up and hollow. Bend your knees up to your chest one at a time. They should be parallel to each other.
- Your arms should be extended alongside your body, palms down and wrists straight, a few centimetres off the floor.

Action
1 Stay zipped throughout and breathe in wide and full, pumping your arms up and down for a count of five, taking them no more than 15 centimetres off the floor. Keep the shoulder blades down, and the fingers lengthening away.
2 Breathe out and pump the arms for a count of five.
3 Repeat ten times.
4 Work up to twenty repetitions, hence the 'Hundred'.

Watchpoints
- Your breathing should be comfortable – do not over breathe. If you feel light-headed take a break.
- As you beat the arms be aware of any unnecessary tension in your neck and keep it released.
- Your shoulder blades should stay down into your back as your arms lengthen away.

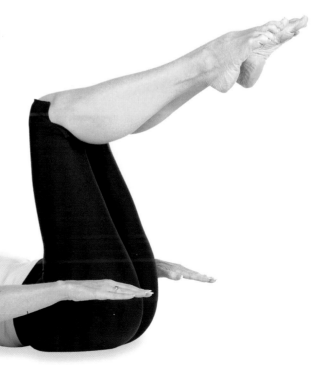

Stage Four

Aim

By adding abdominal training to the breathing technique, you will work the deep neck flexors. Try to keep the superficial neck muscles released.

Warning: please take advice if you have neck, respiratory or heart problems.

Preparation

- Lie in the Relaxation Position (see page 48) with your head on the cushion if it is more comfortable. Zip up and hollow and bring your knees up on to your chest one at a time, keeping the legs parallel.
- Let your arms relax on the mat and slowly roll your head from side to side to release your neck.

Action

1 Breathe in wide and full to prepare.
2 Breathe out, zip up and hollow, then curl the upper body off the floor, remembering everything you learnt for Curl Up (see page 88). Keep the chin gently tucked with the jaw relaxed.
3 At the same time lift the arms off the floor.
4 Soften in the breastbone and release the neck.
5 Zipped and hollowed, start the breathing and pumping action of the arms that you mastered in Stage Three. Breathe in laterally for five beats and out for five beats. Keep directing the shoulder blades down towards the waist.
6 Repeat twenty times until you reach a count of one hundred, then slowly bend your knees to your chest and lower your upper body and head down to the mat.

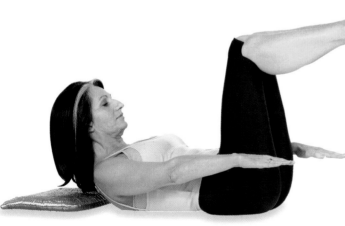

Watchpoints

- Return your upper body to the floor if you feel any strain in your neck.
- To prevent strain and to engage the deep stabilizers, have your chin gently tucked in, but not squashed. Your line of focus should be between your thighs. The back of your neck remains long, the front relaxed.
- You must keep breathing wide into your lower ribcage or you will become breathless. If you do feel breathless, stop at once.
- Keep a sense of width in your upper body. Do not close the shoulders in, keep the upper body open, the breastbone soft.

Stage Five

Warning: please take advice if you have neck, respiratory or heart problems.

Preparation

- Lie in the Relaxation Position (see page 48) with your head on the cushion if it is more comfortable.
- Zip up and hollow, and bring your knees up to your chest one at a time, keeping the legs parallel and the arms by your side.
- Slowly roll your head from side to side to release your neck.

Action

1 Breathe in wide and full to prepare.
2 Breathe out, zip up and hollow, then curl the upper body off the floor, remembering everything you learnt for Curl Up (see page 88). Your chin is gently tucked in and your jaw is relaxed. Keep the breastbone soft and the neck released.
3 Breathe in and then out as, zipped and hollowed, you straighten the legs into the air as high as is comfortable. Keep your legs controlled; do not allow them to fall away or your back will arch – it must stay anchored to the floor. Your feet are softly pointed.
4 Zipped and hollowed, start the breathing and pumping action of the arms that you mastered in Stages One to Four. Breathe in laterally for five beats and out for five beats. Keep the shoulder blades drawn down towards the waist.
5 Repeat twenty times until you reach one hundred, then slowly bend your knees on to your chest and lower your upper body and head down to the mat.

Watchpoints

- Return to the floor if you feel any strain at all in your neck.
- To prevent strain and to engage the deep stabilizers, have your chin gently tucked in but not squashed. Your line of focus should be between your thighs. The back of your neck remains long, the front relaxed.
- You must keep breathing wide into your lower ribcage or you will become breathless. If you do feel breathless, stop at once.
- Keep a sense of width in your upper body. Do not close in the shoulders, keep the upper body open, the breastbone soft.

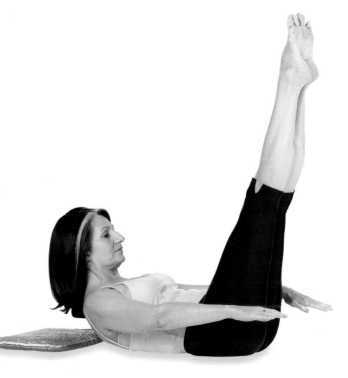

Forward Bend (y)

Aim

This exercise provides a deep opening for the pelvis, lower back and hamstrings. It also gently stimulates the flow of blood to the brain. There are two options – choose the second, simpler variation if you don't have enough flexibility to tackle the first posture.

Warning: be cautious if you suffer from disc problems.

Action

1 From a Standing Posture (see page 51), bring the hands behind the back and clasp one wrist. Take a tiny step forward with the right foot.
2 Keeping the front of the hips relaxed and the shoulder blades down the back, bring the torso forward keeping the upper body straight. Don't be concerned with pushing the head towards the feet.
3 Once in this position, focus on the breath. Follow the movement of the abdomen as it sinks back towards the spine as you breathe out.
4 Find the centre of balance in the feet and release the thighs so the kneecaps drop.
5 Release the ankles and try to let go in the hips and the back of the waist.
6 When you are ready, bend the knees, tuck the tailbone under and roll back up with the shoulders and head last.
7 Now repeat with the left foot forward.

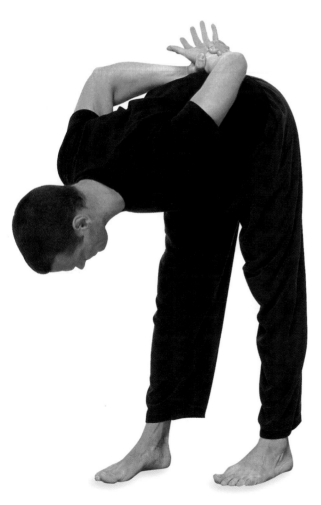

Simple Variation

Rather than clasping your hands behind you, bring them out in front and place them against a wall or chair for support.

Watchpoints

- Don't arch the back – keep dropping the shoulder blades down towards the waist.
- Keep the back of the neck long and the chin gently tucked in.
- Keep a central alignment – don't lean towards one foot or the other.

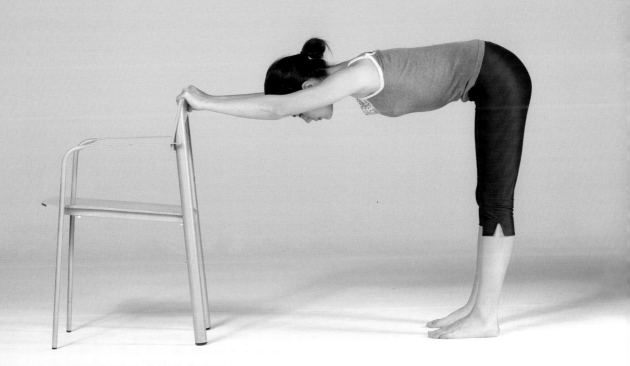

One-legged Seated Forward Bend (y)

Aim

This exercise will help you find foundation in the hips by letting the weight go evenly down through the sitting bones. It stimulates blood flow to the brain and internal organs, cools the body and calms the mind.

Warning: be cautious if you suffer from disc problems.

Equipment

A firm pillow (optional).
A yoga belt or dressing-gown belt.

Preparation

- Sit on the mat with your legs straight out in front of you.
- Make sure you have good postural alignment – ribcage floating above the hips – and use the sitting bones as your foundation.

Action

1 Bring your right foot to rest on the inside of your left thigh.
2 If the right knee has come up off the mat, place the pillow under it for support.
3 Keeping the back straight and with the shoulder blades moving towards the waist, lift up out of the hips and hinge forward as you breathe out.
4 Take hold of your ankle or thigh (or your foot if the body is open enough). If you find this difficult, place the yoga or dressing-gown belt around the arch of the foot and hold on to both ends.
5 When you are seated forward, relax the back of the hips down and lengthen the spine up.
6 Gently tuck the chin in as though you are holding a ripe peach underneath it, elongating the back of the neck.
7 When you are ready, slowly come back up.
8 Repeat on the other side.

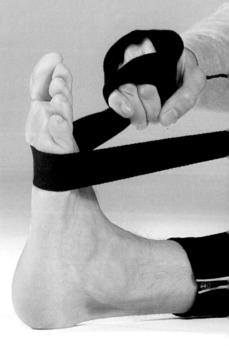

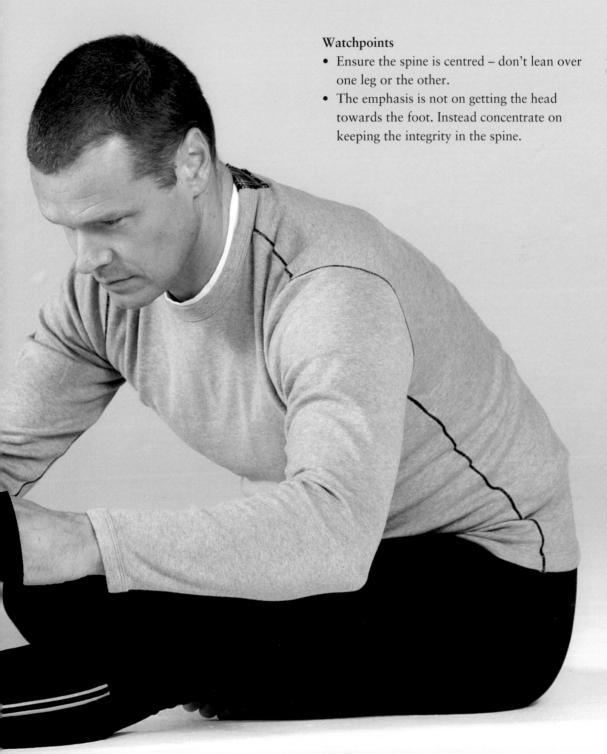

Watchpoints

- Ensure the spine is centred – don't lean over one leg or the other.
- The emphasis is not on getting the head towards the foot. Instead concentrate on keeping the integrity in the spine.

Forward Bend Cobbler (*y*)

Aim

As well as opening the hips, this exercise stimulates blood flow to the pelvic organs, making it good for premenstrual, menopausal and prostate problems.

Warning: be cautious if you suffer from disc problems.

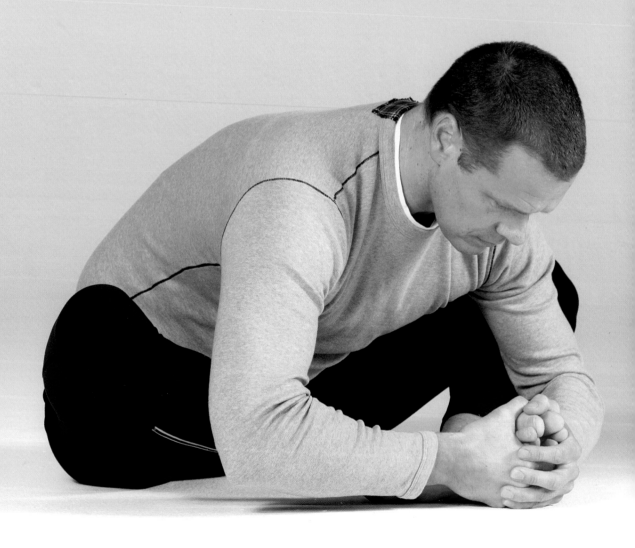

Action

1 Start by sitting on the mat and bring the soles of the feet together, placing the hands behind you with your fingers pointing straight back.

2 Keeping them balanced, release the hips, allowing the gravitational pull to separate the knees. Your weight should be going down evenly through the sitting bones.

3 Use the arms to lengthen the spine, creating space between the ribcage and the hips. Relax the shoulder blades back in the direction of the waist.

4 Open out the front of the chest and relax the shoulders.

5 Tuck the chin in gently to lengthen the back of the neck, as though you are holding a ripe peach beneath it.

6 Once this length has been created, release the hands and bring them on to the feet, holding the toes.

7 Move the feet a few inches forward, keeping the same alignment in the spine as before. You will come forward further as your feet move.

8 Follow the breath for 20 to 30 seconds.

Watchpoints

- If the hips are very stiff, support the knees with a pillow to help the hips release.
- Don't arch the back – keep dropping the shoulder blades down towards the waist.
- Keep the back of the neck long and the chin gently tucked in.
- Keep a central alignment – don't lean towards one foot or the other.

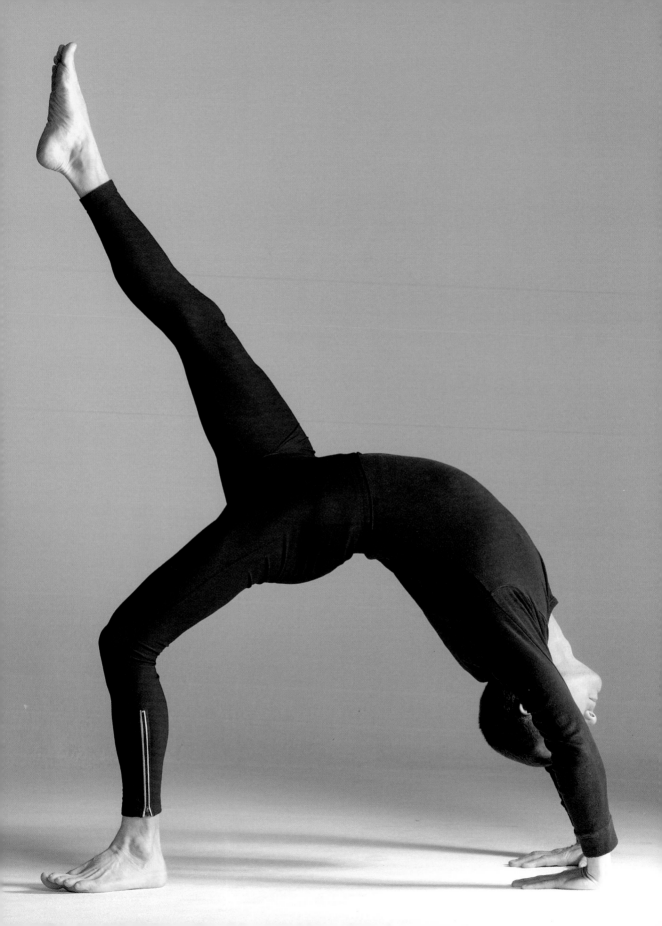

Extension/
Backward Bend

Diamond Press (*p*)

Aim

This subtle exercise has dramatic results and really does help to reverse the effects of being hunched over all day. While encouraging lengthening in and extension of the back, it works the deep neck flexors and the muscles that stabilize the shoulder blades as well as developing an awareness of the scapulae moving on the ribcage.

Preparation

- Lie on the mat face down with your feet hip-distance apart and parallel.
- Create a diamond shape with your arms by placing your fingertips together just above your forehead. If this is not comfortable place the hands further apart.
- Keep the elbows open and the shoulder blades relaxed.

Action

1 Breathe in and lengthen through the spine.
2 Breathe out, zip up and hollow, then pull the shoulder blades down towards the back of your waist. Gently tuck your chin and lift your head 3–4 centimetres off the floor.
3 Keep looking down at the floor so the back of the neck stays long. (Imagine a cord is pulling you from the top of your head.) Really make the connection down into the small of your back – you may have to push a little on the elbows, but think of them connecting with your waist as well.
4 Breathe in and hold the position. Keep the lower stomach lifted, but the ribs on the floor.
5 Breathe out, still zipped, and slowly lower back down. Keep lengthening through the spine.
6 Repeat five times.

Watchpoints

- Keep the lower abdominals drawing back to the spine.

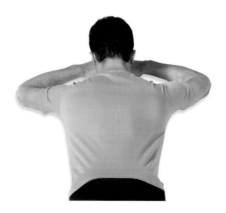

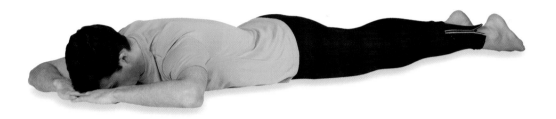

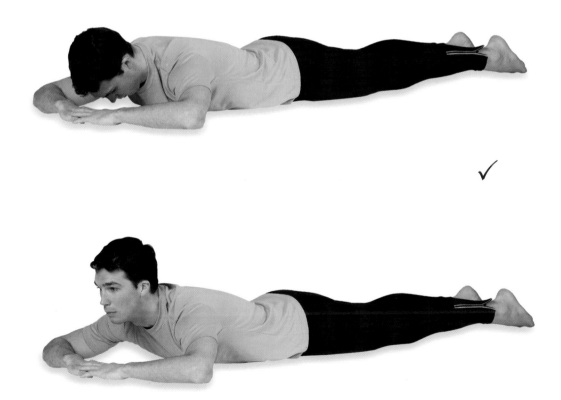

- Make sure that you keep looking down at the floor – tilting your
  head will shorten the back of the neck.

The Dart (Stage Two) (*p*)

Aim

This exercise will create awareness of the shoulder blades and will strengthen the muscles that stabilize them. It will also strengthen the back extensor muscles, and work the deep neck flexors.

Equipment

A small, flat pillow or a towel (optional).

Preparation

- Lie on your front (you may place a small, flat pillow or a small, folded towel under your forehead to allow you to breathe).
- Your arms are down by your sides, your palms are facing up.
- Your neck is long.
- The legs are together, parallel, with your toes pointing.

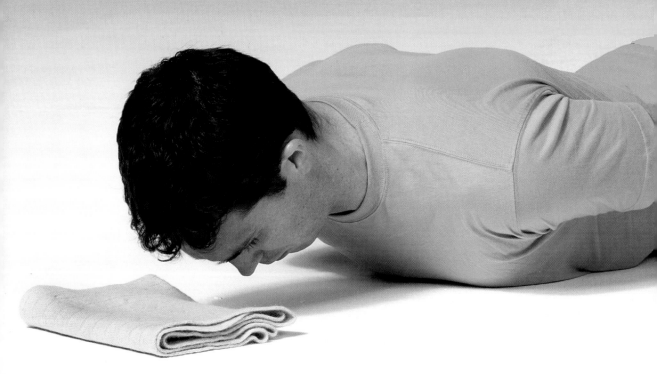

Action

1 Breathe in to prepare and lengthen through the spine, tucking in your chin gently.
2 Breathe out, zip up and hollow, then draw your shoulder blades down into the back, lengthening your fingers towards your feet and turning the hands to face the body. Squeeze your inner thighs together, but keep your feet on the floor and, using the mid-back muscles, slowly raise the upper body from the floor, it does not come up far. Keep looking straight down without tipping your head back.
3 Breathe in and feel the length of the body from the tips of your toes to the top of your head.
4 Breathe out, still zipped, and slowly lower.

Watchpoints

• Keep hollowing the lower abdominals.
• Do not strain the neck – it should feel released as your shoulders engage down into your back. Think of a swan's neck growing out between its wings.
• Keep your feet on the floor.
• Stop if you feel at all uncomfortable in the low back. This exercise can also be done with the feet hip-width apart and the thigh and buttock muscles relaxed.

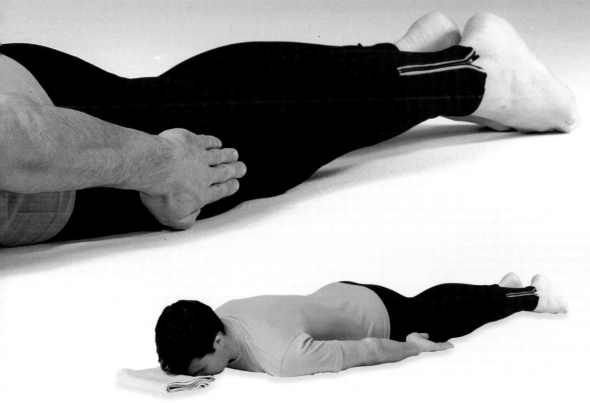

Preparation

Single Heel Kicks (*p*)

Aim

You will improve co-ordination and learn how to extend the back safely and with stability by practising this exercise. It will also gently stretch the abdominals, the quadriceps, strengthen the hamstrings and mobilize and articulate the ankle joints.

Warning: please take advice if you have a back or a knee injury.

Preparation

- This exercise can be carried out either in a sphinx position, with the upper back extended, or with the head down resting on your folded hands. You should be comfortable with the Diamond Press and the Dart before you attempt to extend the back further by doing this exercise in the sphinx position.

- If you are coming up into a sphinx position, place the hands on the floor just wider than shoulder-distance apart, the fingers in line with your ears. Zip up and hollow, and push down on to the forearms to raise the upper body off the floor. Keep the elbows and forearms on the floor. Make sure that your neck remains long, and your shoulders stay well away from the ears and the breastbone. Your pelvis and pubic bone remain on the floor. Stay zipped throughout the exercise.

- You should feel comfortable in this position. If you feel any pinching in your back, come down to the alternative position and rest your forehead on your folded hands. Make sure that your upper back remains open and relaxed.

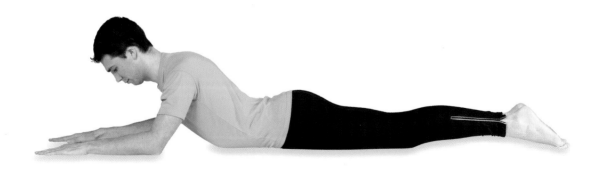

Action

1 Have the legs slightly apart.
2 Zip up and hollow, and point and kick the left foot towards the buttocks. Lower the leg slightly, then flex the foot and kick again.
3 Repeat with the right foot.
4 Repeat eight times with each leg.

Watchpoints

- Breathe normally throughout the exercise.
- If you are in the sphinx position, do not allow yourself to sink down, keep lengthening and zipping and hollowing.
- In either position, make sure that both hips stay in balanced contact with the floor.

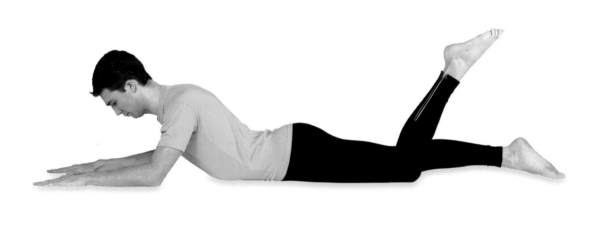

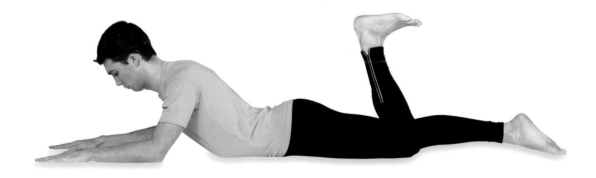

Double Heel Kicks (p)

Aim

A classical Pilates exercise which works
the back muscles, buttocks and hamstrings.
You should be able to do the Dart Stage Two
comfortably before you try this exercise.

Preparation

- Lie on your front in a straight line, resting
  your head to one side. Your legs should be
  together and parallel.
- Clasp your hands behind your back, one
  hand lightly holding the other, with your
  elbows bent. Place the hands as high up the
  back as is comfortable with the elbows
  staying close to the floor.

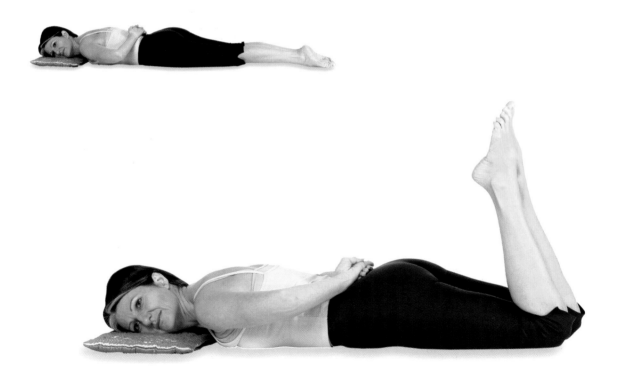

Action

1 Breathe in wide and full to prepare and lengthen from head to toe.
2 Breathe out, zip up and hollow, and stay zipped throughout.
3 Breathe in and quickly kick both feet towards the buttocks three times.
4 Breathe out as you stretch your legs down to the floor.
5 As you lower your feet, move your hands towards them, sliding the shoulder blades down into your back – an action that will bring your upper body up from the floor.
6 Reach down the back with the hands; your feet are back on the floor.
7 Breathe in. Slowly lower the upper body back to the floor, turning the head to the other side and bring your hands back to the starting position and kick three times.
8 Repeat five times.

Watchpoints

• Your lower abdominals should support the spine at all times.
• Remember everything you learnt while doing the Dart on page 65. Keep your neck long and your shoulder blades lengthening away.
• Imagine a piece of string attached from your hands to your feet – this will help the action to be smooth and flowing.

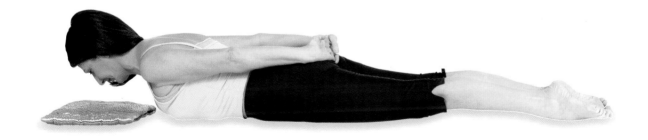

Extended Cobra (*y*)

Aim

In yoga, backbends are used to open the chest and heart areas as well as release negative emotions and encourage a sense of well-being. They stimulate the nervous system, most of the major organs and promote suppleness in the spine and core. Always treat backbends with great respect – remember, the saying 'to bend over backwards for someone' means to do something that is not easy – and counterbalance them with the Resting Child position (see page 118) to calm the nervous system, open out the vertebrae and release the back muscles. The Extended Cobra opens out the middle of the back to reduce excessive curvature of the thoracic spine and breaks up tension in the shoulders. It is a safe precursor to other, more strenuous backbends.

Warning: those with back problems should show caution.

Action

1 Lie face down on the mat with your forehead resting on the floor. Your elbows are bent and close to the body. Your hands are about 30 centimetres out in front of you with your middle finger pointing forwards. Point your toes.

2 Lift the head and chest and straighten the arms so that the elbows are off the floor. Leave the abdomen and the bottom of the ribcage touching the floor so that you work the middle of the back.

3 Tuck your toes under your heels and lift the knees and thighs off the floor so that you are resting on your abdomen, pubic bone, hips and toes.

4 Keep the buttocks soft and drop the shoulder blades down to the waist.

5 Follow your breath for 20–30 seconds, then lengthen and move back into the Resting Child position.

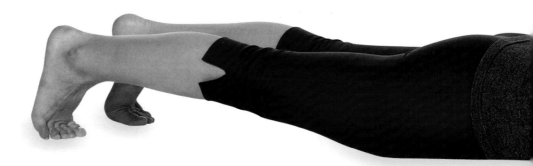

Watchpoints

- Keep the shoulder blades moving down towards the waist.
- The chin should be gently tucked in, as if holding a ripe peach.
- Find your foundation in the hips – relax and release the weight through the front of the hips.

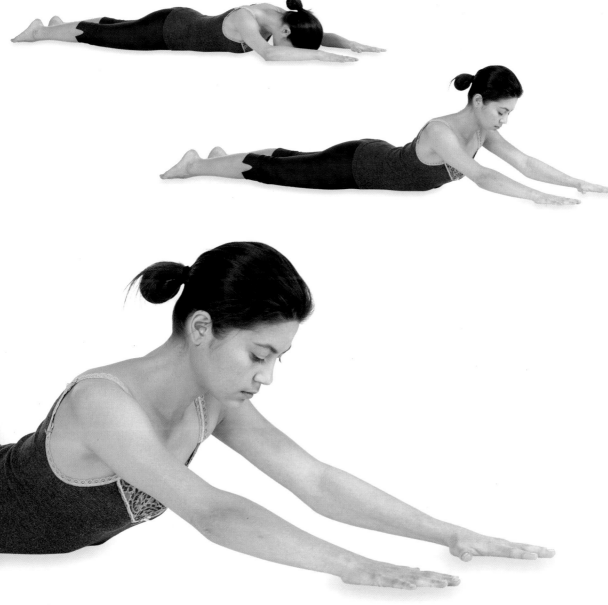

Full Cobra (*y*)

Aim

This exercise increases strength in the back and arms, keeps the spine supple and opens out the chest, encouraging deep, full breathing. It also stimulates the kidneys and adrenal glands.

Warning: avoid this exercise if you have any spine or back problems.

Preparation

- Lie face down with your forehead resting on the mat. Bend your elbows and have them close to the body. The hands are in a line and alongside the centre of the chest.

Action

1 Open the hands from the centre of the palm, with the middle finger pointing forwards.
2 As you breathe out, lift the chest and shoulders off the mat. Lift up, out of the hips and keep the chin tucked well in to elongate the spine.
3 Once you have reached as far as you can, bring the head up tucking the chin in so you look towards the horizon.
4 Keep the head in line with your upper back to form a smooth curve. This will avoid closing up the back of the neck, waist and throat.
5 The foundation should be in your hands, hips and thighs.
6 The front of the chest should be open to release the shoulders.
7 Bend your elbows and bring them in towards your ribcage.
8 Breathe for 20–30 seconds then come down to lying.
9 Follow with Resting Child (see page 118).

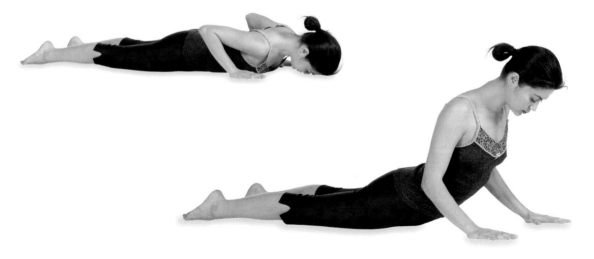

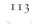
Watchpoints

- Come up with a snake-like movement – remember it's called the cobra, not the banana!
- This exercise is often taught with the head back, but by tucking in the chin the spine lengthens and the deep abdominals are pulled back to support it.
- Keep the shoulder blades dropping down towards the waist to open out the front of the chest.
- Don't push up into the shoulders. The emphasis is on releasing the back of the neck and shoulders, not straightening the arms.

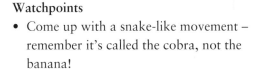

Locust (y)

Aim

This exercise increases strength in the upper and lower back, stimulates the sex glands and reduces gas in the lower abdomen. Once you can do the first two stages successfully, try the more complex variation.

Warning: avoid this exercise if you have any spine or back problems.

Equipment

A folded towel.

Preparation for both stages

- Place a folded towel across the centre of your mat to give your hip bones some extra padding.
- Lie face down with your forehead on the mat and your arms alongside your body, palms facing up.
- The feet should be hip-distance apart.

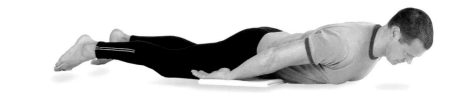

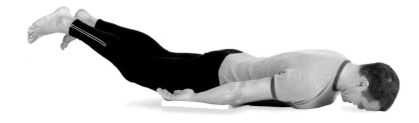

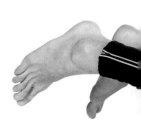

Action for Stage One

1 As you breathe out, bring your chest and shoulders off the mat.
2 The chin should be tucked in to keep the back of the neck long.
3 Slide the shoulder blades down towards the waist to open the chest.
4 Stay in this position for as long as is comfortable, then release down.
5 Rest.

Action for Stage Two

1 With the toes pointing, lift the thighs, knees and feet off the mat as you breathe out.
2 Keep the ankles, shoulders and back of the neck relaxed.
3 Rest.
4 Now combine these two movements, lifting for as long as is comfortable and using the centre of the body as your foundation.
5 Follow with Resting Child (see page 118).

Watchpoints for Stages One and Two

• Keep the back of the neck long – don't bring the chin up too far.
• Keep the hips released.

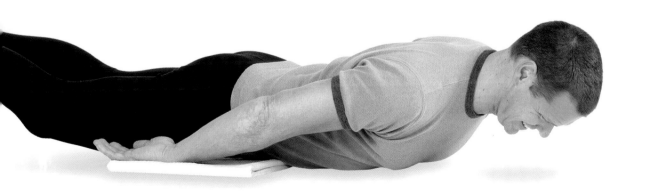

Bridge (*y*)

Aim

Ideal for strengthening the core muscles in the spine, hips and thighs, the Bridge also opens the chest, heart and lungs, promoting full breath.

Warning: avoid this exercise if you have any spine or back problems.

Preparation

- Begin in the Relaxation Position (see page 48). Place both feet on the mat, hip-distance apart and parallel, with the heels under the knees.

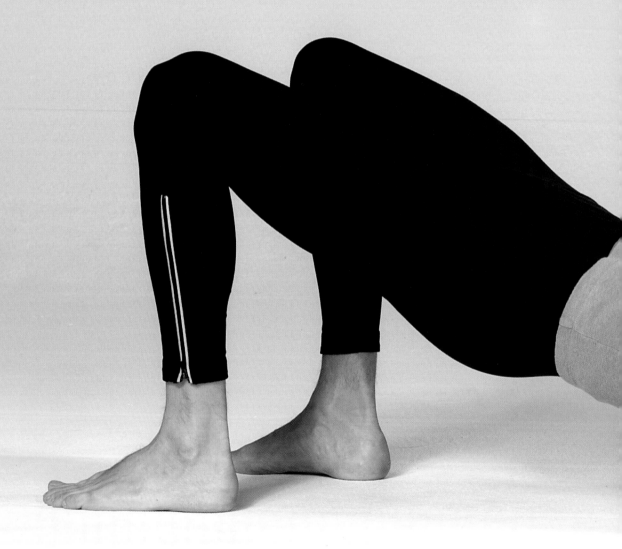

Action

1 Bring the arms out to the side, palms facing up. Keeping the arms on the floor bend them at the elbows and point the fingers.
2 As you breathe out, move the knees forward keeping the feet on the floor, so that the hips lift off the mat as high as possible. Keep the shoulders soft.
3 You should be in a straight line from the knees to the shoulders.
4 Follow the breath for 20–30 seconds, or until the body starts to feel tense.
5 Bring the hips down and hug the knees towards the chest.

Watchpoints

• Have the knees above the feet, if not closer.
• The foundation should be in the soles of the feet and shoulders.
• Keep the thighs, buttocks and front of the hips soft without dropping the body.

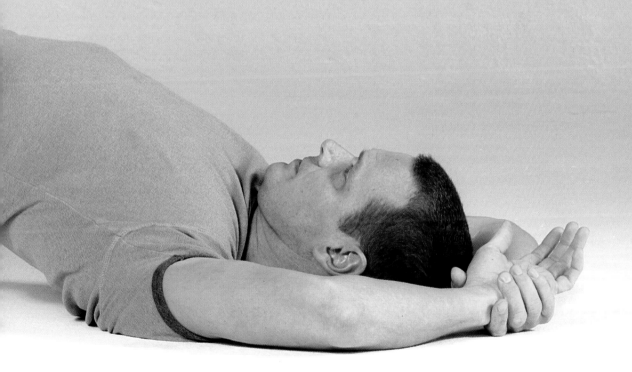

Resting Child $(p+y)$

Aim

As this is the position that the spine develops in while growing in the womb, it gives the body natural alignment and is a great way to stretch out after any demanding backbend. This will open out your sacral, lumbar, middle and upper spine as well as your hips and inner thighs. It will also allow the head and neck to rest and give you control of your breathing in a relaxed position. In Pilates, this is called the Rest Position; in yoga it is known as the Child's Posture. The only difference is the positioning of the arms – choose which version is right for you.

Warning: avoid this exercise if you have a knee injury. You can curl up on your side in the foetal position instead or place a pillow behind your knees.

Equipment

A pillow or a towel (optional).

Action

1 Come on to all fours and bring your feet together, keeping your knees slightly apart.
2 Keeping the hands still, slowly move back and down towards your buttocks until you are sitting on your feet. Your forehead should touch the floor if possible, if not use a pillow or folded towel to rest on.

For a Pilates Stretch:

1 Relax in this position, leaving the arms extended in front of you. Feel the expansion of the ribcage as you breath deeply into the back.
2 To deepen the stretch for the inner thighs, spread your knees further apart and think of sinking your chest towards the ground.

For a Yoga Stretch:

1 Draw your arms behind you and relax them by your side. Position the hands alongside the feet, with the palms facing upwards.
2 Follow the breath.

To finish

1 As you breathe out, zip up and hollow, then drop your tailbone down bringing the pubic bone forward, and slowly came up to a kneeling position, uncurling vertebra by vertebra.
2 Bring your head up last, keeping the shoulders relaxed.

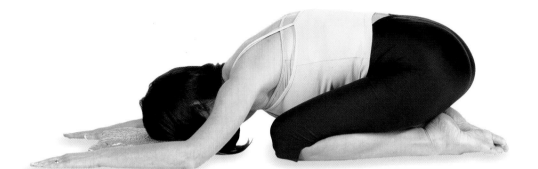

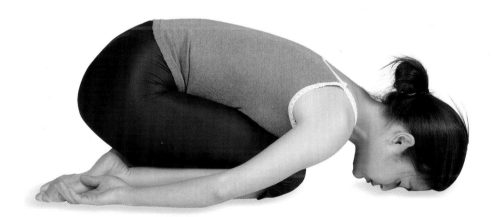

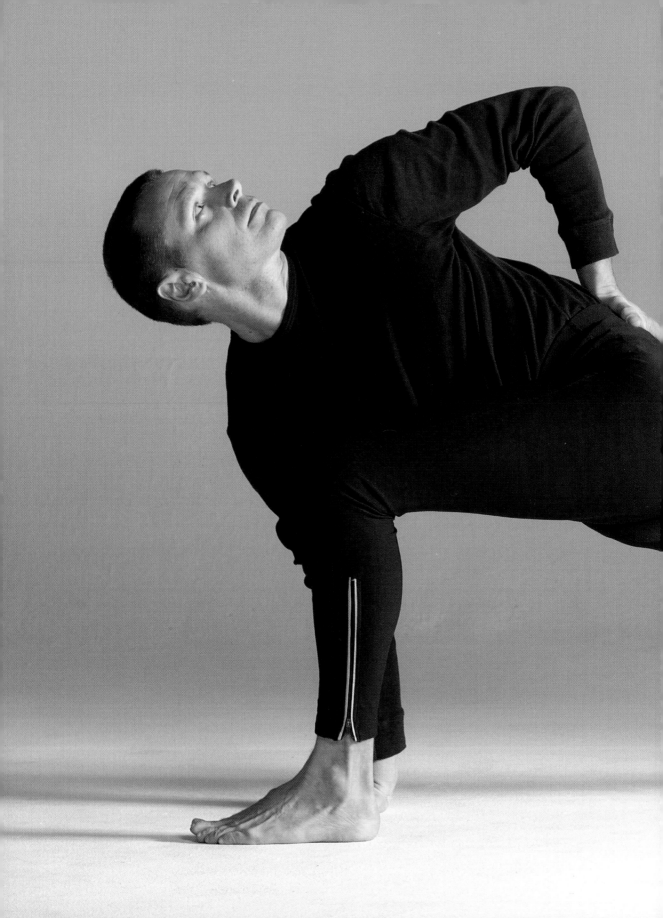

Rotation / Spinal Twist

Hip Rolls (p)

Aim

To give the spine stability as you rotate it, as well as really toning the waist muscles (obliques).

Warning: take advice if you have a back injury, especially any disc-related problems.

Preparation

- Lie in the Relaxation Position (see page 48) but with your feet together.
- Place your arms out to the sides at shoulder height, palms upwards and allow the body to lengthen and widen.

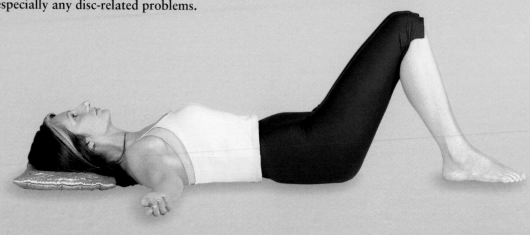

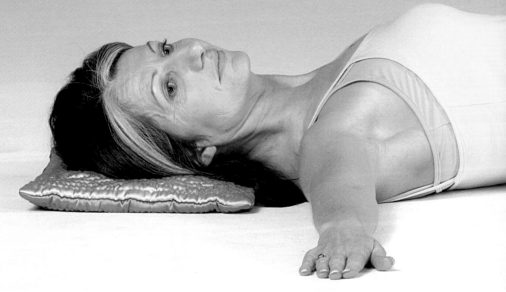

Action

1 Breathe in wide and full to prepare and, as you breathe out, zip up and hollow. Roll your head in one direction and your knees in another.

2 Turn the palm you are looking at down. Keep your opposite shoulder on the mat and only roll a little way to start with – you can go further each time if it is comfortable.

3 Think of rolling each part of your back away from the ground in turn – buttocks, small of the back, waist and ribcage.

4 Breathe in, still zipped. As you breathe out use your core strength to bring the knees back into the starting position, along with your head. As you come back to the middle, turn your hand back up.

5 Repeat eight times in each direction.

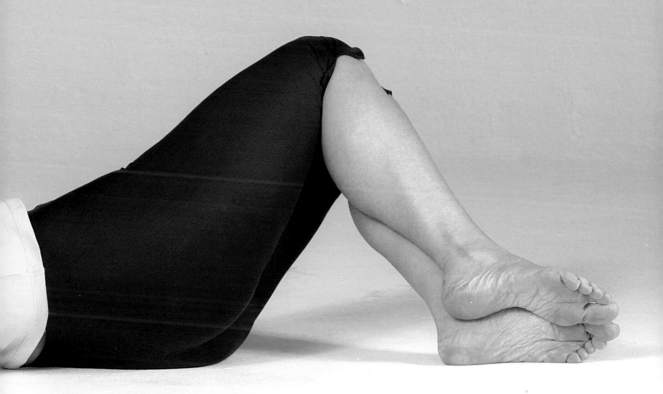

Hip Rolls (p) (intermediate)

Aim

When you have mastered the version of Hip Rolls on page 122 and your abdominals are stronger, attempt this more challenging rotation.

It really works the obliques, which help define your waist.

Equipment

A tennis ball.

Preparation

- Lie on your back, arms out to the side and palms up.
- Zip up and hollow and raise your knees one at a time towards your chest so they are above your hips. Your thighs will be at right angles to your body, feet softly pointed.
- Place the tennis ball between your knees.

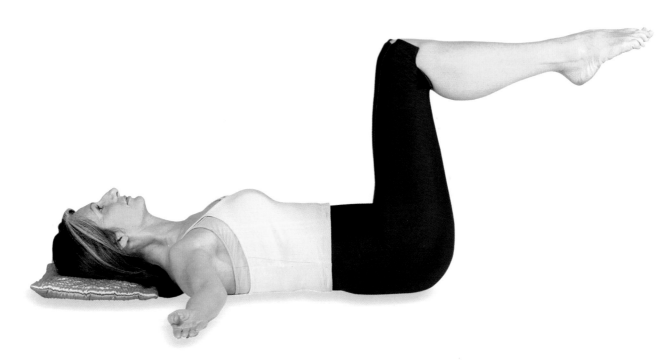

Action

1 Breathe in wide and full to prepare then, as you breathe out, zip up and hollow and slowly lower your legs (a little way at first) toward the floor on your left side, turning your head to the right and turning the right palm face down.

2 Keep the right shoulder down on the ground and the knees in line.

3 Breathe in and breathe out, still zipped, then use this strong centre to bring your legs back to the middle. The head returns to the centre too.

4 Repeat up to eight times to each side, going a little further each time but always keeping the opposite shoulder blade down into the back. Think of each part of the back coming off the floor in turn – the buttock, the waist, the lower ribcage – and then returning in reverse order – the back of the ribcage, the waist, the buttock.

Watchpoints

- Keep the opposite shoulder firmly down on the floor.
- Keep the knees in line and don't go too far unless you can control the movement.
- Use the abdominals – feel as though you are moving the legs from the stomach.
- Control the movement and don't allow the weight of your legs to pull you over.
- Do not force the neck the opposite way, allow it to roll comfortably and keep it released and lengthened.

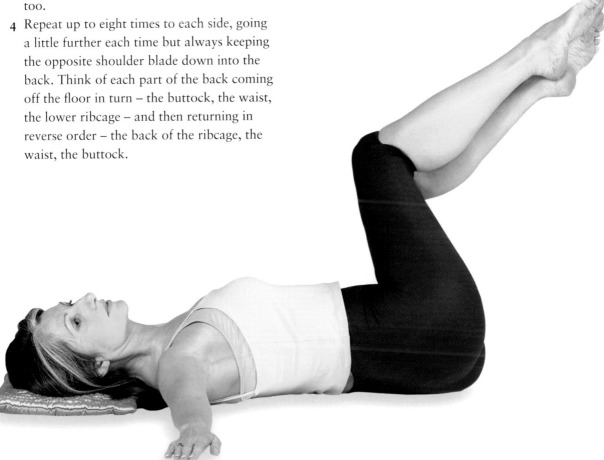

Bow and Arrow (p)

Aim

This wonderful exercise opens the upper body and teaches you to turn while lengthening. The action is similar to drawing a bow!

Preparation

- Sit tall with your legs bent in front of you – if you have the flexibility, stretch your legs out straight – and make sure that you are sitting on your sitting bones.
- Hold your arms out in front of you at shoulder height, palms facing down.
- Your shoulder blades are down into your back and your neck is released.

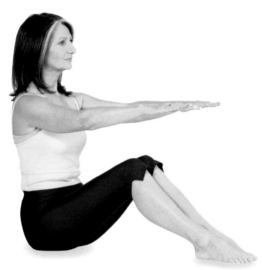

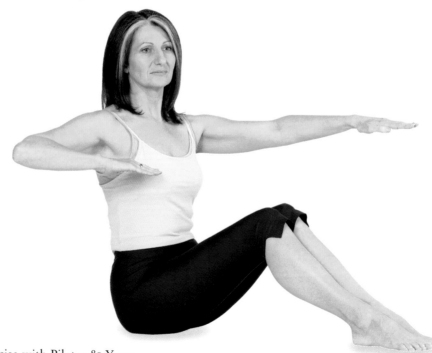

Action

1 Breathe in wide and full and lengthen through the spine.
2 Breathe out, zip up and hollow, then stay zipped throughout.
3 Breathe in and fold one hand in towards your chest. The elbow stays up in a line with the shoulder.
4 Still on the in breath, follow the action through as you turn the upper body, unfolding the arm as it straightens out behind you. Your head follows the action but stays in a line with your spine.
5 Your upper body is now open.
6 Breathe out and bring the arm back to the front in a wide circle.
7 Repeat 5 times to each side. You can help the rotation through the body by imagining that your straight arm is being pulled by a piece of string.

Watchpoints

- Keep lengthening up through the spine – don't allow the waist to sag.
- Keep your arms at shoulder height.
- Keep the shoulder blades down into your back.
- Keep the movements slow and flowing.
- Keep the knees and feet together – this ensures your pelvis stays square.

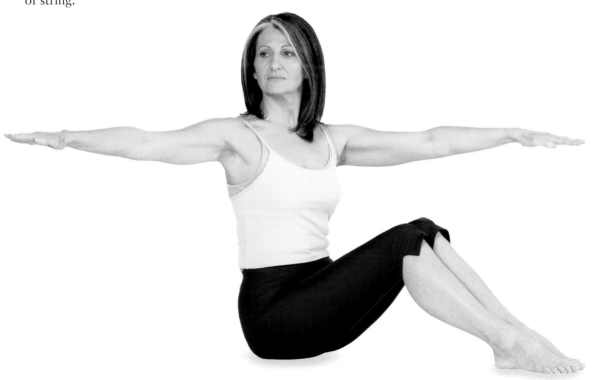

Waist Twist (*p*)

Aim
Use this exercise to learn rotation of the spine with stability and length. You may also like to try this exercise breathing in as you turn – some people find they get a better routine on the in breath.

Warning: consult your practitioner if you have a disc-related injury.

Preparation
- Begin in the Standing Posture (see page 51) and hold your arms out to the side. If they tire, lower them.

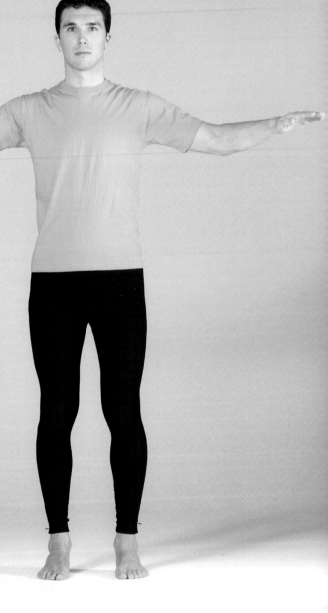

Action

1 Breathe in as you lengthen up through the spine.
2 Breathe out and zip up and hollow. Keeping your pelvis square and facing forward, gently turn your upper body around as far as is comfortable. Your head will turn also but only go as far as you can keep your pelvis square and still.
3 Breathe in as you return to centre.
4 Repeat up to ten times to each side.

Watchpoints

- Do not allow the shoulders to creep up around the ears – keep the shoulder blades down into the back.
- Try to keep the weight evenly balanced through both buttocks and on both feet.
- Do not turn the head too far. It should move naturally, balanced on top of the spine.
- Try not to tilt forward with one shoulder, stay central.
- Pay close attention to keeping the correct pelvic alignment. If you find your pelvis moving, stand in front of a table or the back of a chair with your thighs just touching it – this will give you an idea of when you twist the pelvis.

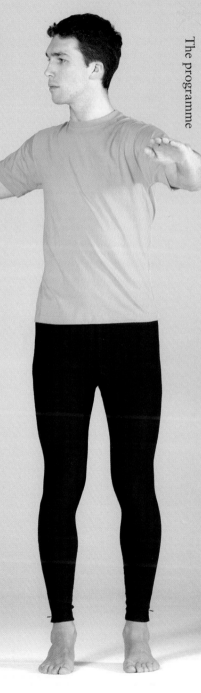

Standing Spinal Twist (*y*)

Aim

Twists are powerful postures. They relax tight back muscles, release toxins and improve the circulation of blood and oxygen to the nervous system. They massage the internal organs and intestines to promote good bowel function and can help to relieve minor aches and discomforts in the back after long sitting, forward or back bending. It is important to rotate both sides of the torso for an equal amount of time and rest afterwards. Rotations keep the deep spinal muscles supple and release tension in the spinal column. They also stimulate blood flow to the spinal cord and tone the large intestine.

Warning: those people with spinal problems should show caution.

Preparation

- Begin in the Standing Posture (see page 51), with your feet parallel and hip-distance apart.
- Place the right hand on the top of the chest, palm down.
- Place the left hand on the middle of the back, palm facing outwards. When this area of the back starts to relax, the front of the chest begins to open as it lifts from the inside.

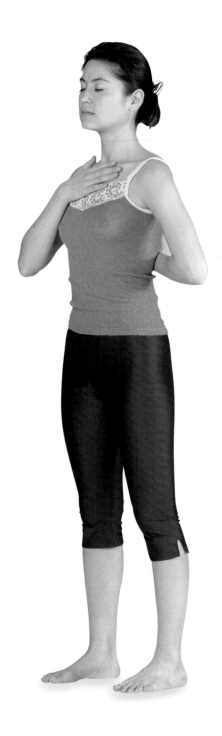

Action

1 Imagine your hips are against the front of a table to help you stabilize.
2 Start to move as you breathe out, rotating to the left, open side.
3 Keep the hips facing forwards.
4 Keeping the neck long, gently tuck the chin as you bring it round to the left shoulder.
5 Breathing out, move back to the centre.
6 Before you rotate to the left, find your neutral alignment again.
7 Change your hand position and repeat on the other side.

Watchpoints

- Try not to use the shoulders as a lever. Rotate using the muscles in the back.
- Don't over-rotate – the skeletal system can move further than the organs within the body, so while over-stretching may feel good, you're causing tension within the body.
- If you start to feel a pull in the ankles and the soles of the feet curl, the hips have moved out of their stable position.

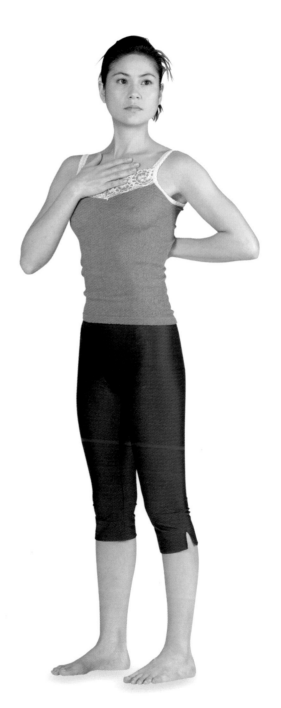

Seated Spinal Twist (y)

Aim

Rotations keep the deep spinal muscles supple and release tension in the spinal column. They also stimulate blood flow to the spinal cord and tone the large intestine.

Warning: those people with spinal problems should show caution.

Preparation

- Sit in a comfortable cross-legged position.
- Use the same alignment as for standing, but find your foundation in the sitting bones to stabilize the hips.

Action

1. Release the shoulder blades to find alignment between the hips and the ribs. Keep the spine long.
2. Bring the right hand behind the hips. Lightly place the fingertips on the mat and relax the right shoulder. Place the left hand on the ankles.
3. Start to rotate from the abdomen as it moves back to the spine while you breathe out.
4. As you rotate, bring the left hand and place it on the right knee.
5. Keeping the neck long, gently tuck the chin as you bring it round to the right shoulder.
6. Breathing out, move back to the centre.
7. Before you rotate to the left, find your neutral alignment again.
8. Repeat on the other side.

Watchpoints

- Try not to use the arms and shoulders as levers – this causes tension in the spine.
- Rotate from the abdomen.
- Keep the area below the shoulder blades soft and relaxed and the spine long. The rotation comes from the middle of the back – if it is tight, it won't rotate.

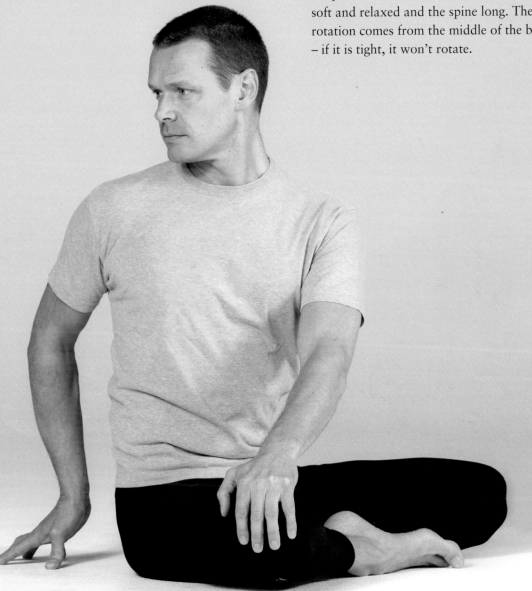

Lying Down Spinal Twist (*y*)

Aim
As for Seated Spinal Twist.

Warning: those people with spinal problems should show caution.

Equipment
A plump pillow (optional).

Preparation
• Lie on your back and gently hug your knees to your chest.

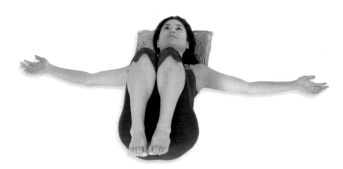

Action
1 Keeping the knees still, extend the arms out to the side and rest them on the floor, palms facing the ceiling.
2 Stabilizing the shoulders on the mat, breathe out and bring both knees down to the left until they touch the mat. If necessary, use a plump pillow under the knees for support.
3 Release the left hand and relax it on the right knee.
4 Release the right hip and shoulder to open out the space between the waist and the hips. Keep the chin gently tucked in and look towards the ceiling.
5 As you breathe out, follow the movement back towards the spine (see yoga breathing on page 33), releasing the deep muscles along its length.
6 Breathing in, bring the knees back up to the centre.
7 Breathing out, repeat on the other side.

Watchpoints
• Always keep the opposite shoulder open and resting on the mat.

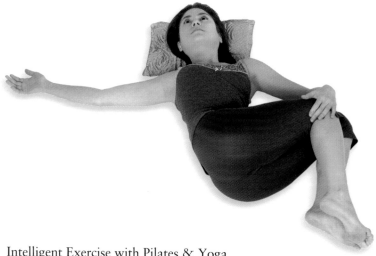

Simple Variation

If you feel too much tightness to bring the
knees down all the way, try this variation.
Instead of hugging the knees to the chest,
place the feet together on the floor to begin
with. Stabilize and then take both knees
down to the left, keeping both feet
and knees on top of each other.

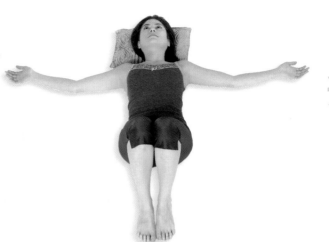

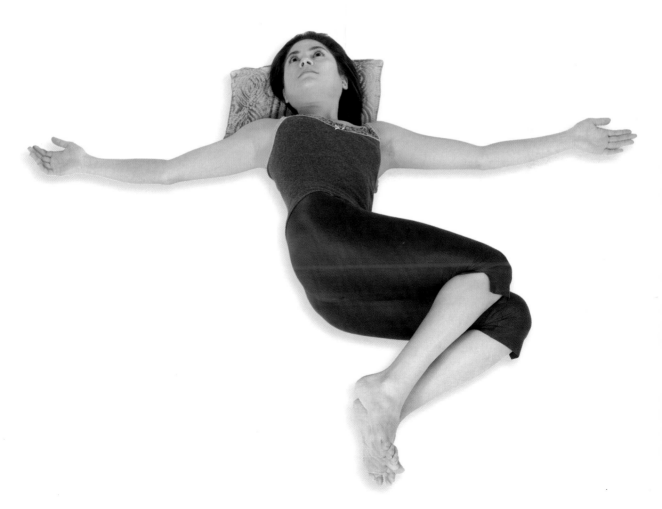

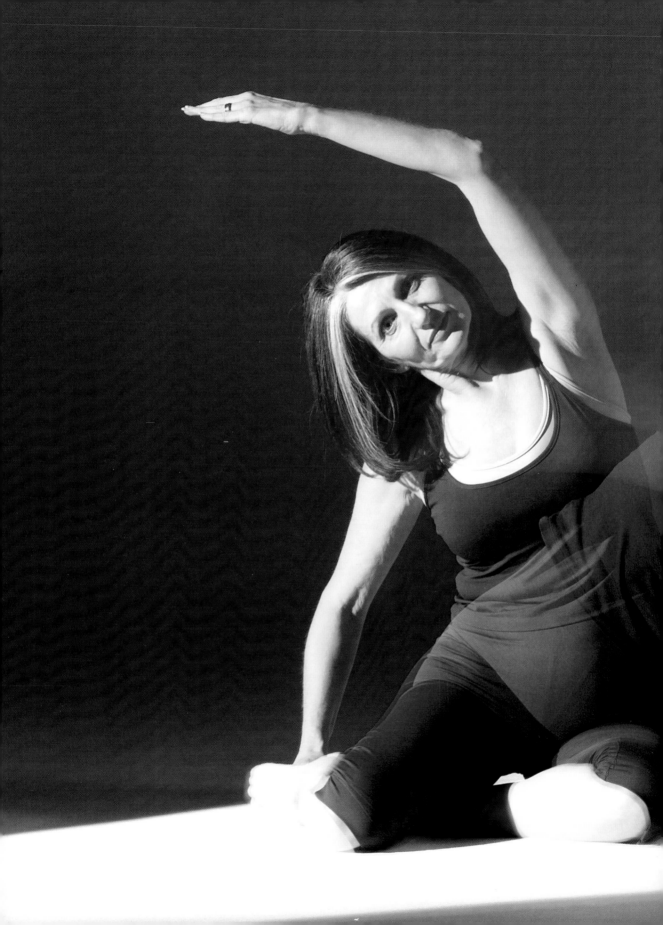

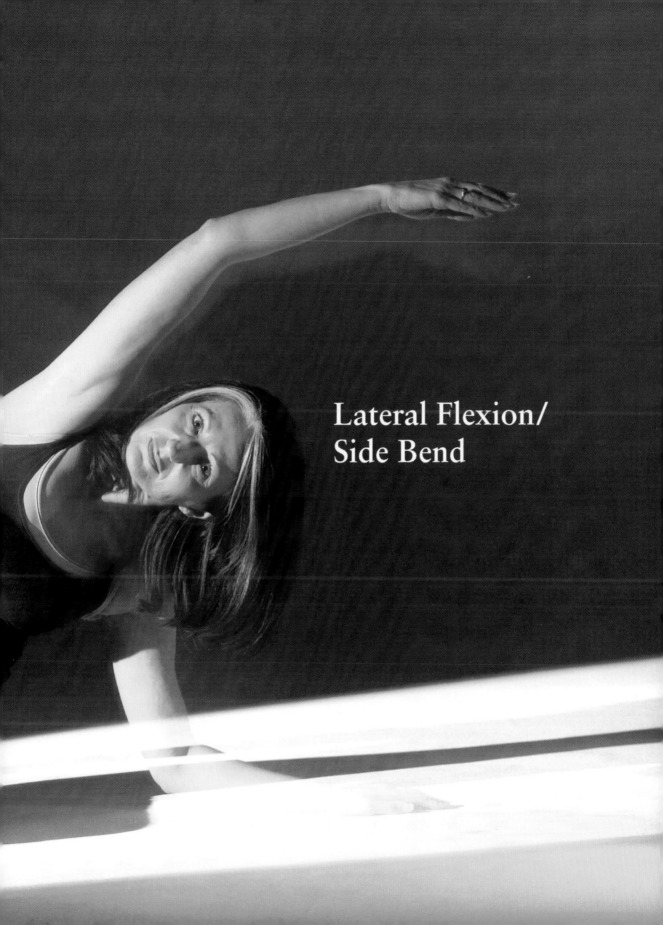

Lateral Flexion/
Side Bend

Simple Standing Side Reach (*p*)

Aim

Try this to stretch and tone the side muscles while achieving a sense of length and stability. It always feels good.

Preparation

- Stand with your feet wider than your hips, with the feet parallel.
- Release the knees slightly and remember your good postural alignment from the Standing Posture (see page 51). The arms should be down by your sides, hands resting on your thighs.

Action

1 Breathe in wide and full, then lengthen up through the spine as you raise one arm.
As your arm floats up think of your shoulder blades moving down to start with and then widening outwards. Keep your neck and upper shoulders soft.
2 Breathe out, zip up and hollow. Lengthening upwards, reach towards the opposite top corner of the room. Your other arm should slide down the outside of the thigh.
3 Open and feel the distance between the ribcage and your pelvis. Make sure that you go directly to the side and not forwards or backwards, keeping your focus straight ahead.
4 Breathe in and keep lengthening upwards. Breathe out, still zipped, then slowly return to the centre, lowering your arm.
5 Repeat five times on each side, keeping the pelvis central.

Watchpoints

- Be careful not just to bend sideways, collapsing the waist. You must keep lengthening upwards.
- Keep your pelvis central.
- Watch the angle of the head – keep it on top of the spine, looking forwards.

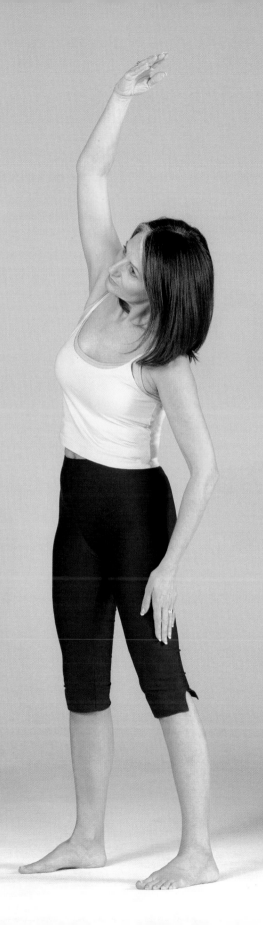

Mermaid (p)

Aim
A great exercise for stretching out your waist and strengthening the upper body.

Warning: take advice if you have back or sacroiliac joint problems.

Preparation
- Sit on the floor facing forwards with your legs bent and your knees out to your left-hand side. Have them a comfortable distance away from your body, in a line with each other. Have your weight on the left hip.
- Lightly clasp the front of your right shin with your right hand.
- Even though you are sitting at an angle, keep lengthening up through the spine.

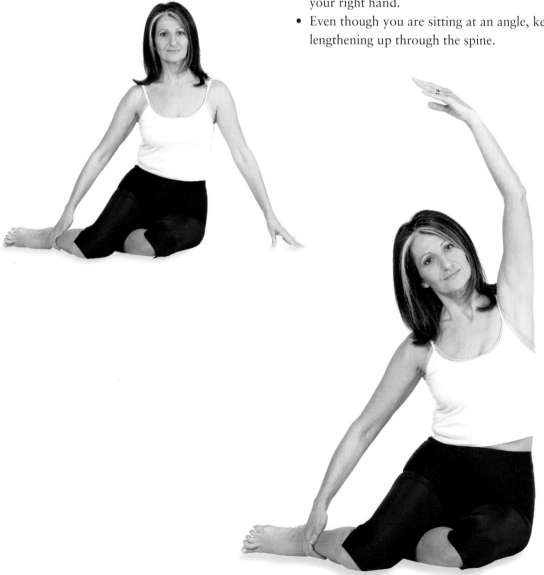

Action

1 Breathe in wide and lengthen up through the spine.
2 Breathe out, zip up and hollow (stay zipped now), and float your left arm up. Your palm faces inward.
3 Breathe in wide and full and lengthen up.
4 Breathe out and reach the arm across to the right aiming for the top corner of the room. Reach through the fingertips, feel the stretch between your ribs and your hips along your left side. Keep the distance between your ears and your shoulders.
5 Breathe in wide and come back to centre.
6 Breathe out and lower the left arm to the floor, coming on to the elbow if you can. Raise the right arm to reach across to the left, palm facing down.
7 Enjoy the stretch along your right side. Keep your right hip down to increase the stretch.
8 Breathe in and push up on the left elbow to return to the starting position. Use the momentum of coming up to carry you through on the out breath, stretching to the right once again.
9 Repeat 5 times on each side.

Watchpoints

• Keep the movement slow and flowing, a bit like a reed bending in the wind.
• Try to stretch directly to each side in the same plane, without tilting forward or back.
• Remember everything you learnt in Floating Arms about good upper-body movement.

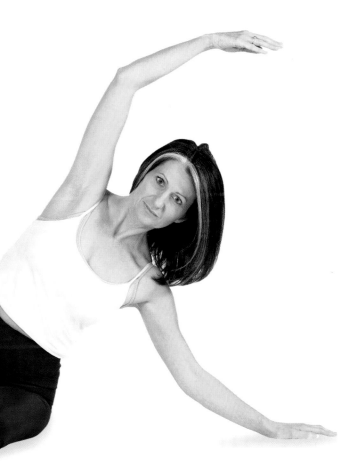

Side Bend (*p*)

Aim
Great for overall strength – think long and strong.

Warning: avoid this exercise if you have shoulder, arm or neck problems.

Preparation
- Lie in a straight line on your left side, with your legs stretched out in a line with your body.
- Prop up your upper body on the left elbow and hold your right hand softly in the air. Take the right leg and place it in front of the other. Put your right foot close to the ankle of the left. The right foot should be pointing forward.

Action
1. Breathe in wide and full to prepare and lengthen through the spine.
2. Breathe out, zip up and hollow (stay zipped now), and lift your right hip up towards the ceiling by pushing into your right foot.
3. At the same time float the right arm up and over your head to reach across to the top corner of the room. Squeeze your inner thighs together.
4. Breathe out and slowly lower the whole body to the mat circling the right arm back down.
5. Repeat up to five times on each side.

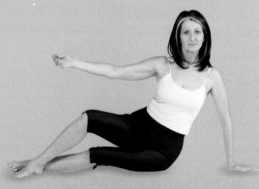

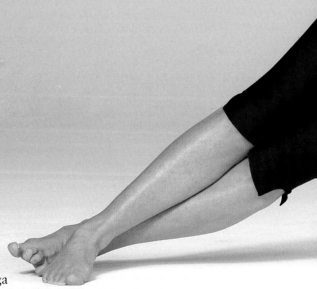

Watchpoints

- When you have lifted your body from the mat, try to keep your pelvis and spine in neutral. Do not let the pelvis roll forwards.
- It helps to imagine a large thick strap wrapped around your hips and lifting you up towards the ceiling.
- Try not to push into the shoulders and arms. They will be working but the weight is on the front foot.

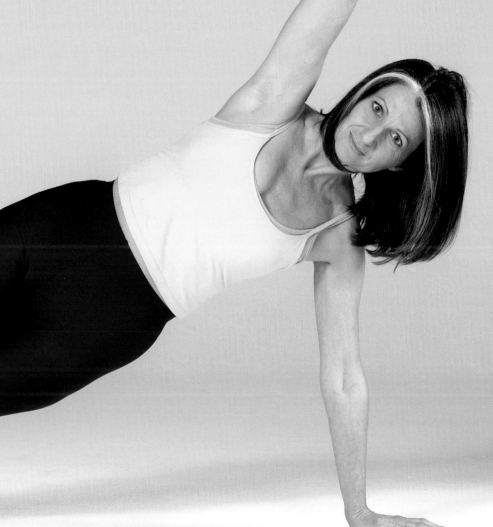

Seated Side Bend (*y*)

Aim

A great posture for releasing the hip, opening the side ribs, shoulders and side, and elongating the spine. During this exercise it's important to get a sense of the abdomen being lifted out of the hip girdle – an action just like zipping up and hollowing.

Warning: those people with back and disc problems should show caution.

Preparation

- Sit comfortably in a crossed-legged position.
- Find your alignment and use the sitting bones as your foundation.

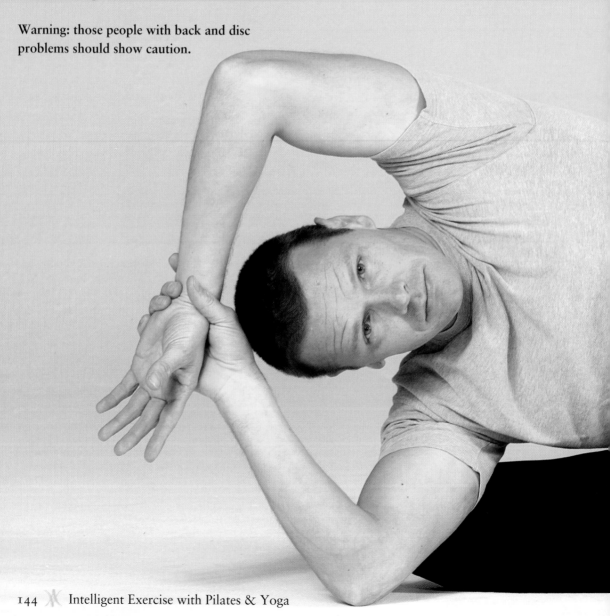

Action

1 Place the right elbow down on the mat just in front of the right knee.
2 If you can, try and rest the shoulder down on to the right knee.
3 Bring the left arm above the head and clasp the left wrist with the right hand. The foundation has now moved to the outside edge of the right hip and thigh.
4 Keep the head in neutral, chin tucked in gently, eyes looking forward.
5 As you breathe out, release the left side of the waist to allow the space between the hips and ribs to open out.
6 Come back to the centre and repeat on the other side.

Watchpoints

- Imagine that the upper body is between two walls. Keep the front of the chest flat so that it doesn't collapse.

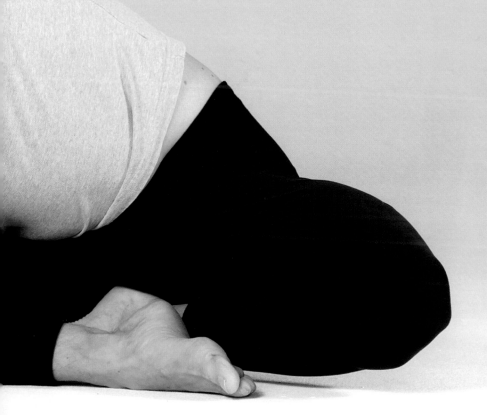

Standing Side Bend (*y*)

Aim

This exercise opens the chest, shoulders and side of the body as well as opening and strengthening the hips and improving digestion.

Warning: those people with back and disc problems should show caution.

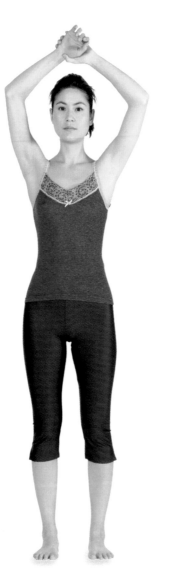

Preparation

- Begin in the Standing Posture (see page 51), then cross the right foot over the front of the left, keeping the heel up and the toes flexed.

Action

1 Bring the arms above the head and clasp hold of one wrist with the other hand.
2 Taking the weight on to the right foot, breathe out and start to come down on the left side, bending from the waist. Be careful not to collapse the stomach.
3 Release the right hip and open the right side of the abdominals, all the way up to the shoulder.
4 Your head should be looking down towards the heel of the right foot.
5 Hold for as long as you feel comfortable.
6 Come back to the centre as you breathe out.
7 Come down to the right side and take the right hip out over the right foot. As you transfer the weight, the left hip goes out to the side and the left side stretches out.
8 Hold for as long as you feel comfortable.
9 Come back to the centre.
10 Cross the left foot over the right one and repeat on other side.

Watchpoint

- Stay in line – don't twist the body or lean forwards or backwards.

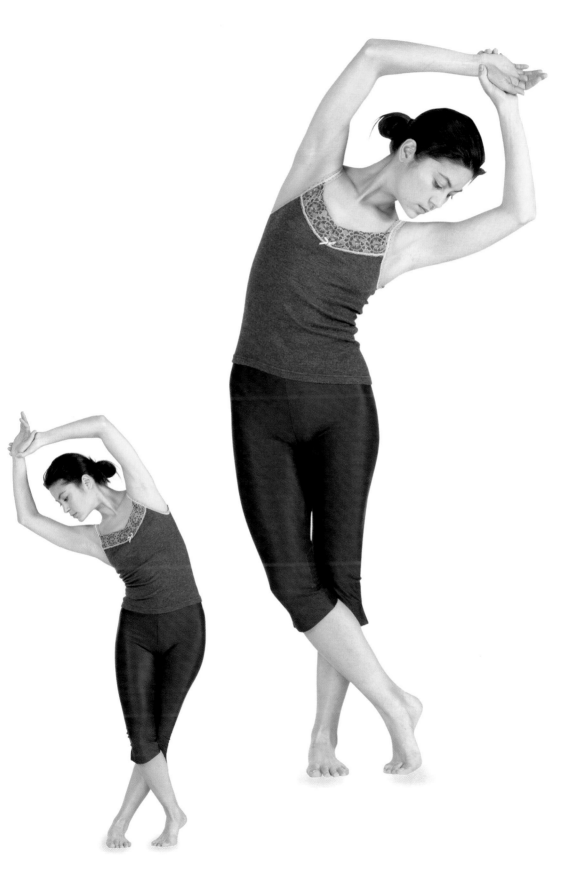

Triangle (*y*)

Aim

To open the chest, shoulders and sides of the body as well as opening and strengthening the hips and improving digestion.

Warning: those people with back and disc problems should show caution. If you suffer from lower-back problems, a stiff neck or shoulders, do not extend your arm upwards during this exercise. Instead, do the exercise alongside a wall for correct alignment and support.

Preparation

- If you are having difficulties with alignment, stand at right angles to a wall, with your left side nearest to it.
- From the Standing Posture (see page 51), take a large step forward with the right foot. Turn the back foot out at 45°.

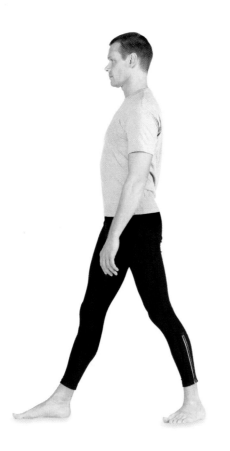

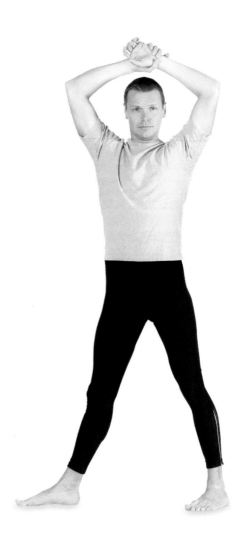

Action

1 If you can comfortably manage it and have achieved good alignment, bring your hands above your head and clasp hold of one wrist.
2 Rotate the upper body and hips to the left (so you are facing flat to the wall). The hips should now be at a right angle to the right foot.
3 Bend your right knee slightly.
4 As you breathe out, bring the right hand on to the knee or ankle of the right leg. Place the left hand gently on the back of the hips.
5 The left shoulder should be pointing up towards the ceiling. The chest and hips are parallel to the wall in front of you.
6 Keep the chin tucked in, the back of the neck long and the eyes looking straight ahead. Gently rotate the neck and look towards the ceiling.
7 If you want to extend the left arm, move your fingertips towards the ceiling. If you want to take the posture further, slowly straighten your right leg.
8 Breathing out, come up and repeat on the other side.

Watchpoints

- There is a tendency to lean forward in this position. Stay centrally aligned and let yourself rest back.
- Keep the back of the hips as open and turned out as possible.
- Soften between the shoulder blades to allow the shoulder blades to drop and open the chest.
- If your arm is extended up, don't use it as a lever to pull back – this jams the spine.
- If you straighten the front leg, don't over-extend the back of the knee.

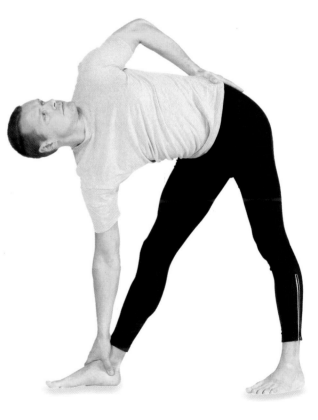

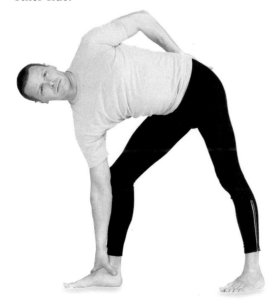

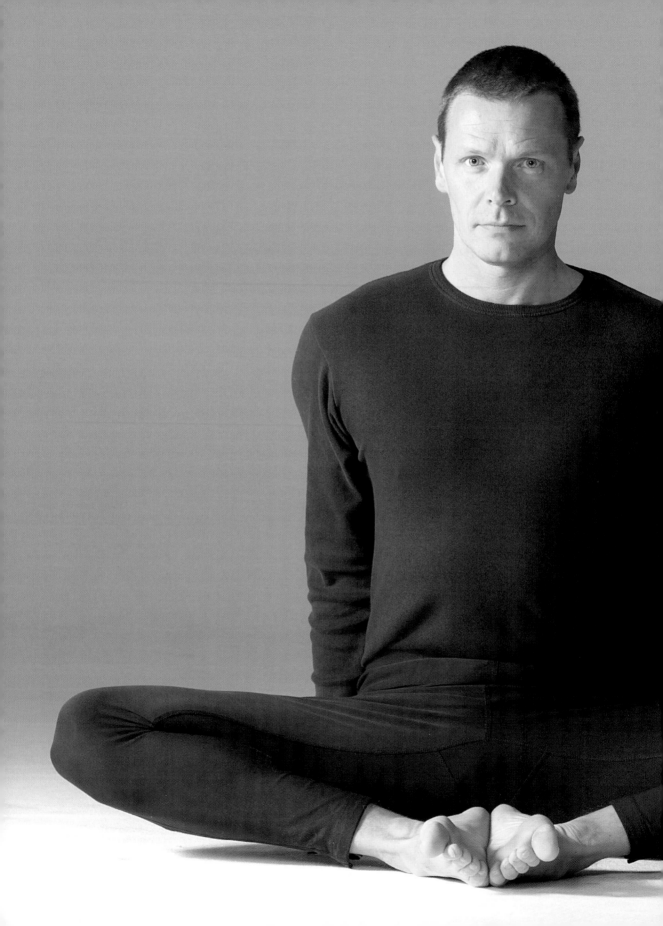

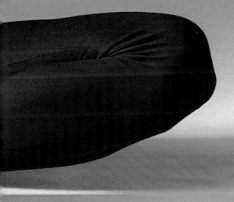

The Pelvis and Hips

*Most of us spend far too much time sitting down,
which unfortunately is one of the worst positions
for the health of the spine and also for the balance
of the muscles around the pelvis and hips. Shortened
hamstrings, hip flexors and adductors and weakened
gluteals affect the angle of the pelvis and can also
contribute to restricted movement around the hips.
The following exercises help to open the hips,
balance the muscles and promote good mobility.*

Zigzag Against a Wall (*p*)

Aim

Ideal for mobilizing the hips, knees and ankle joints.

Equipment

A small flat pillow.

Preparation

- Lie on the floor about half a metre away from a clear wall space.
- Your hips should be square to the wall, your head resting on a small flat pillow.
- Place the feet, together, on to the wall.
- Check that your pelvis is in a neutral position.

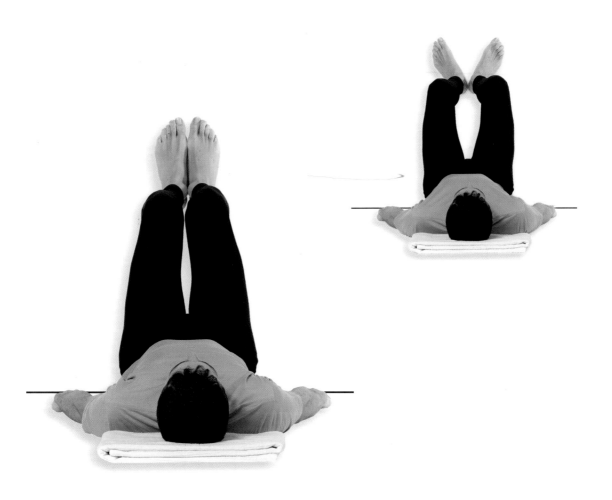

Action

1 Slide your toes apart as far as they will go, keeping the heels together.

2 Keeping the balls of the feet still, slide the heels apart as far as they will go.

3 Continue zigzagging the feet in this way, making certain they stay flat on the wall.

4 You should be transferring the weight of the feet alternately through the heels and through the balls of the feet.

5 Zigzag until the feet refuse to turn any more. The legs will be as wide as you can comfortably open them without changing your pelvic alignment. Then zigzag back together again. Repeat three times.

Watchpoints

• Check that the level of your feet has not dropped and that both feet are at the same height.

• Try not to lift the feet off the wall. You are pivoting alternately on the balls and heels of the feet but letting them slide.

• Keep neutral.

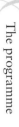

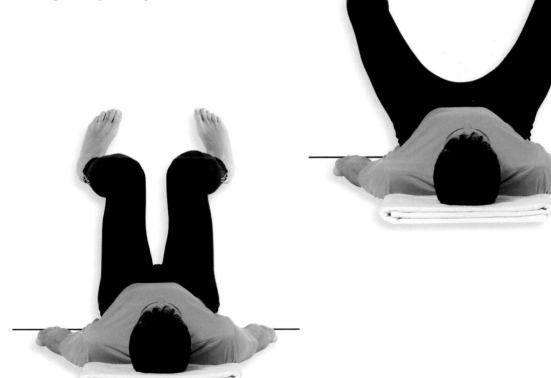

Side-lying Quadricep and Hip Flexor Stretch (*p*)

Aim

This exercise will stretch out the quadricep muscles that run along the front of the thigh and the hip flexors as well as maintaining good alignment of the torso by using the waist muscles and the shoulder stabilizers. It will also lengthen and iron out the front of the body, especially around the front of the hips, which can get very tight if you sit all day.

Notice the position of the pelvis. We actually ask you to tilt the pelvis backwards (to north), losing neutral. This is because there is a danger with this exercise that you may arch the back and stress the lumbar spine so it is better to play safe and tuck slightly. Also by tilting the pelvis you can isolate the hip flexor muscles.

Warning: please take advice if you have a knee injury. You may need to use a belt to hook over the foot so that there is less pressure on the knee, or you may need to leave this exercise out.

Equipment

A belt and a pillow (optional).

Preparation

- Lie on your side with your head resting on your extended arm (you may like a flat pillow between the head and the arm to keep the neck in line).
- Have the knees curled up at right angles to your body – your back should be in a straight line, but with its natural curve.
- Line all your bones up on top of each other – foot over foot, knee over knee, hip over hip and shoulder over shoulder.

Action

1 Breathe in wide and full to prepare and lengthen through the spine.
2 Breathe out, zip up and hollow, and bend the top knee towards you taking hold of the front of the foot if you can reach it (use the belt if necessary).
3 Breathe in and check your pelvic position. You would normally be in neutral in this position but, if you prefer, tuck your pelvis under to north (see above).
4 Breathe out, zip up and hollow, then gently take the leg backwards to stretch the front of the thigh. Do not arch the back but keep the tailbone lengthening away from the top of your head.
5 Hold the stretch for about twenty seconds, working the waist the whole time and keeping the length in the trunk.
6 After twenty seconds slowly release by bending the leg back and then letting go. Keep zipping throughout.
7 Repeat twice on each side.

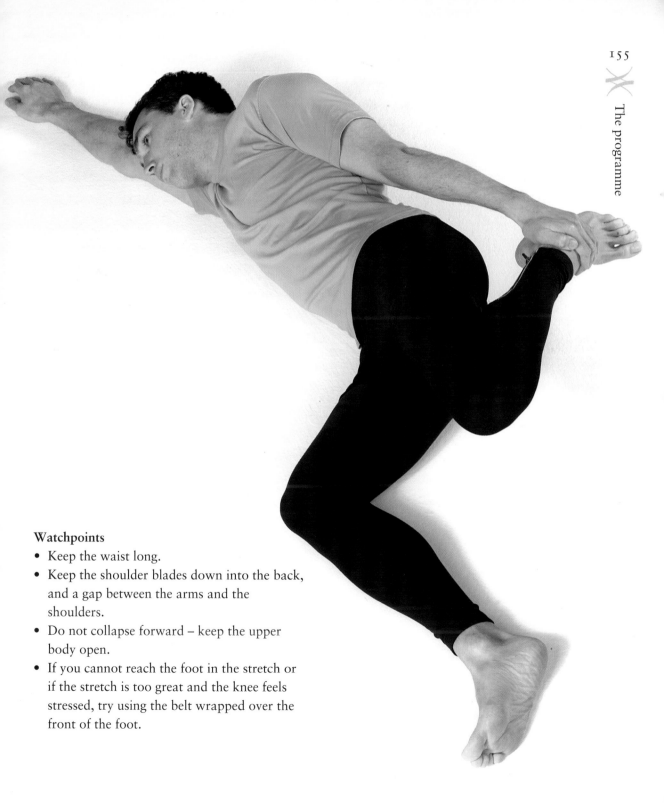

Watchpoints
- Keep the waist long.
- Keep the shoulder blades down into the back, and a gap between the arms and the shoulders.
- Do not collapse forward – keep the upper body open.
- If you cannot reach the foot in the stretch or if the stretch is too great and the knee feels stressed, try using the belt wrapped over the front of the foot.

Hip Flexor Stretch (p)

Aim

If you sit all day, it is likely that your hip flexor muscles will shorten and this will affect the angle of your pelvis, pulling it anteriorly. Use this exercise to lengthen the hip flexors gently.

Action

1 Lie in the Relaxation Position (see page 48) and breathe in wide and full to prepare.
2 Breathe out and zip up and hollow. Keeping that sense of hollowness in the pelvis, hinge the right knee up to your chest, dropping the thighbone down into the hip joint.

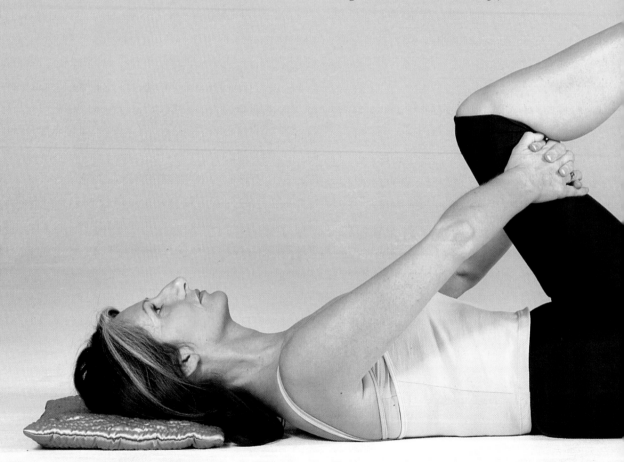

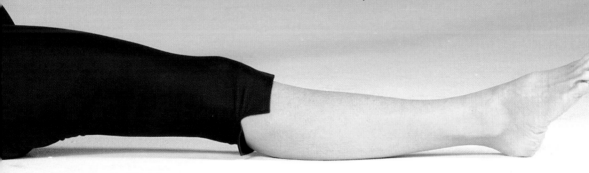

3 Breathe in as you clasp the left leg below the knee or at the lower part of the thigh. If you have knee problems clasp the leg under the thigh rather than below the knee so that the joint is not compressed.

4 Breathe out, still zipped, and stretch the right leg along the floor. Your lower back should remain in neutral. If it arches, bend the right knee back up again a little. Hold this stretch for five breaths.

5 Breathe in as you slide the leg back.

6 Breathe out and zip up and hollow, as you lower the bent leg to the floor, keeping the abdominals engaged.

7 Repeat twice on each side, keeping your shoulders relaxed and down.

Watchpoints

• Check the position of the upper body: elbows open, breastbone soft, shoulder blades down into the back, neck released.

• Are you in neutral?

Cobbler (y)

Aim

As well as calming and settling the mind, this exercise releases the hip joints and opens out the adductor muscles. It also strengthens the back and improves circulation through the hips and legs.

Warning: if your have back problems sit with your back against the wall for support.

Equipment

A pillow (optional).

Action

1 Start by sitting on the mat and bring the soles of the feet together, in front of the groin.
2 Place the hands behind you with your fingertips pointing backwards, palms face down.
3 Release the hips, allowing the gravitational pull to separate the knees. Your foundation should be in your sitting bones.
4 Use the arms to lengthen the spine, creating space between the ribcage and the hips. Relax the shoulder blades back in the direction of the waist to open the front of the chest and shoulders.
5 Tuck in the chin to lengthen the back of the neck and look towards the horizon.
6 Once you've created this length, you can release the hands and bring them on to the feet, holding the toes. Keep the same alignment in the spine as before.
7 Follow the breath and stay in this position for as long as is comfortable.

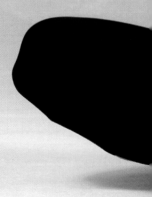

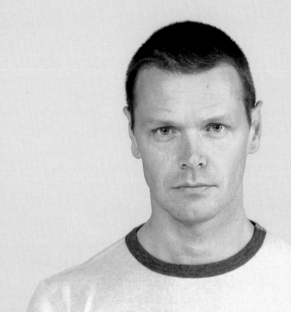

Watchpoints

- If the hips are very stiff, support the knees with a pillow to help the hips release.
- Don't arch the back – keep dropping the shoulder blades down towards the waist.
- Keep the back of the neck long and the chin gently tucked in.
- Keep a central alignment – don't lean towards one side or the other.

King Pigeon (*y*)

Aim

Use this posture to open the outside edge of the front leg, as well as the front of the hip in the back leg. It will also stimulate the blood flow to the pelvis.

Warning: avoid this exercise if you have knee problems.

Preparation

- Sit cross-legged, then take the left leg behind you into a comfortable bent position.
- Come on to the outside edge of the right hip.
- Have the right knee pointing straight out in front of you with the leg bent at right angles and the foot flexed. The centre of the foot should be opposite the knee.
- Let the right hand sit alongside the right thigh for support, while the left hand rests on the left leg.
- Try to find alignment in the spine above the hips as much as possible.
- Keep the shoulder blades down, the neck long and look towards the horizon.

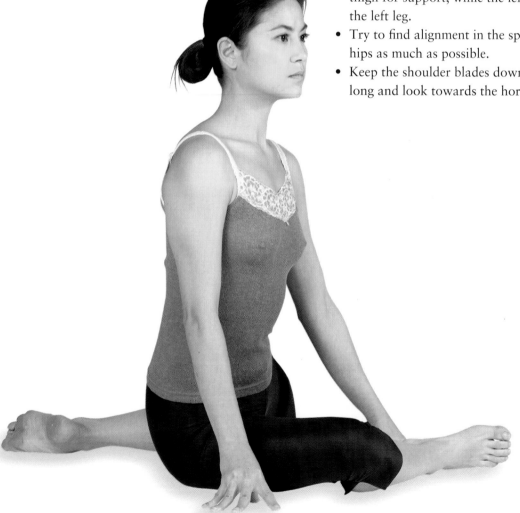

Action

1 Breathing out, come forward from the abdomen.

2 Lay the spine along the length of the right thigh if possible – you don't have to come all the way down. Put the right arm flat on the floor and come on to the elbow to support yourself if necessary.

3 If you are comfortable, extend the left leg back along the mat behind you.

4 Breathing out, allow the right hip joint to deepen as it releases. Stay in this position for as long as is comfortable.

5 Come up to sitting as you breathe out again and repeat on the other side.

Watchpoints

- You should be quite comfortable with the support of the ground and thigh, but don't become sleepy in the position. Keep your awareness in the hip and use the end of each exhalation to find a deeper release.

- The foundation will be in the right hip and thigh – let the weight go down through them.

- Keep the spine long over the leg – try not to round the back.

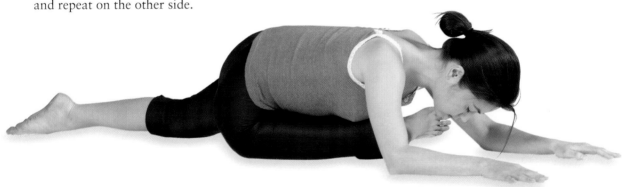

Crescent Moon (*y*) (*advanced*)

Aim

This exercise develops flexibility in the front of the groin and hips, while opening the chest and shoulders and elongating the spine. As this is an advanced exercise, we have also given you a simple version.

Warning: those people with knee and back problems should show caution.

Equipment

A folded yoga mat or a towel (optional).

Preparation

• Start from the Downward Facing Dog position (see page 180).

Action

1 Move the right foot forward between the hands. Your fingertips and toes should be in line.

2 Drop the left knee back on to the mat (use a folded yoga mat or towel for extra padding if necessary).
3 Come up, with the torso above the hips. Keep the weight forward so the right knee is over the heel of the right foot.
4 Bring the hands above the head and clasp hold of one wrist.
5 Let the shoulder blades drop down towards the waist to open the front of the chest.
6 Point the toes of the left foot behind you to open the foot.
7 Breathing out, release the hips and allow the torso to be pulled down with gravity. Do not hold this position for too long.
8 Bring the hands alongside the feet, sweep the right foot back so you come into the Downward Facing Dog position again.
9 Rest and allow the hips to settle then repeat on the other side.

Preparation and
finish position

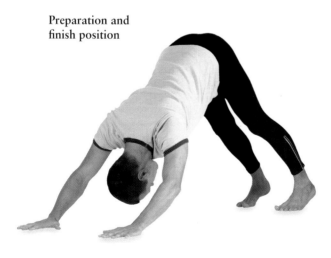

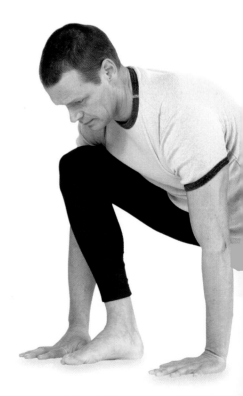

Simple Variation

Watchpoints
- The foundation should be in the front foot.
- You should not be lunging or sinking, but releasing the hips in order to move deeper into the stretch.

Have the back knee closer to the front foot so that the knee and hip are in line, the front leg is at right angles and the heel is under the knee. Place the hands above the head then tuck the tailbone underneath the hips to open out the thigh of the back, supporting leg.

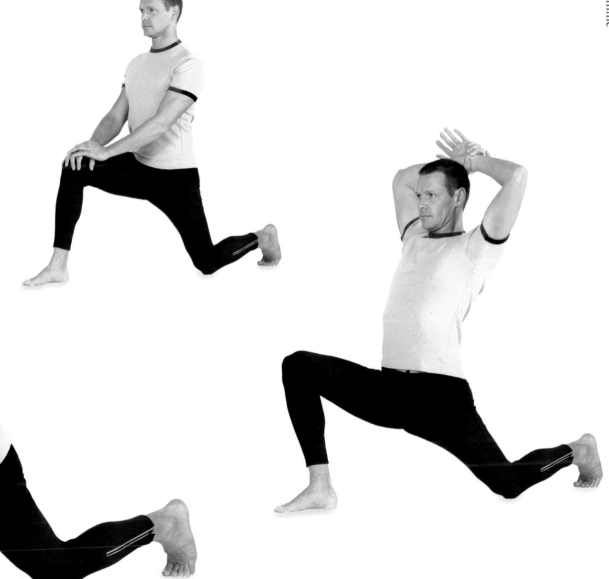

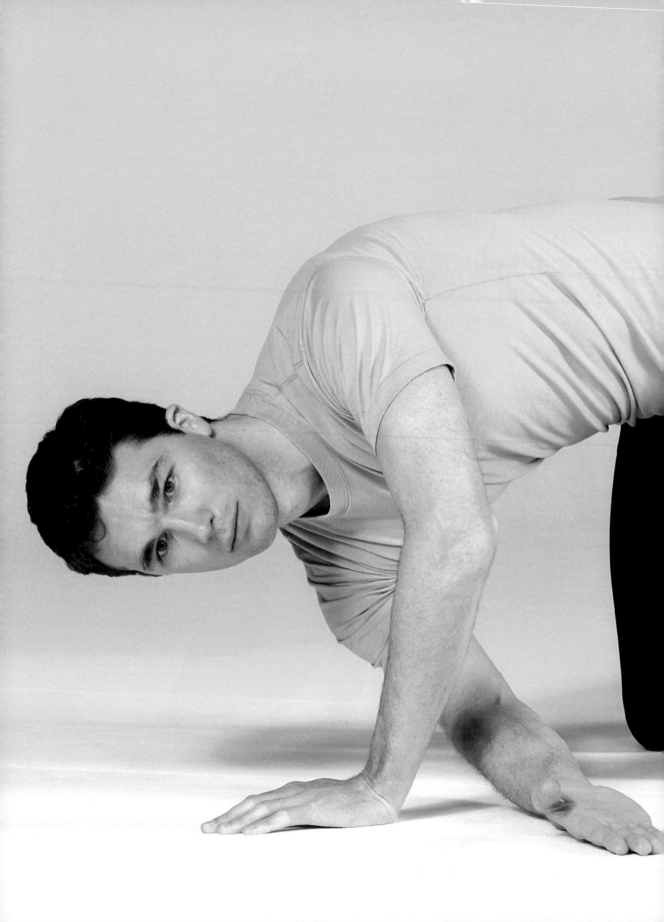

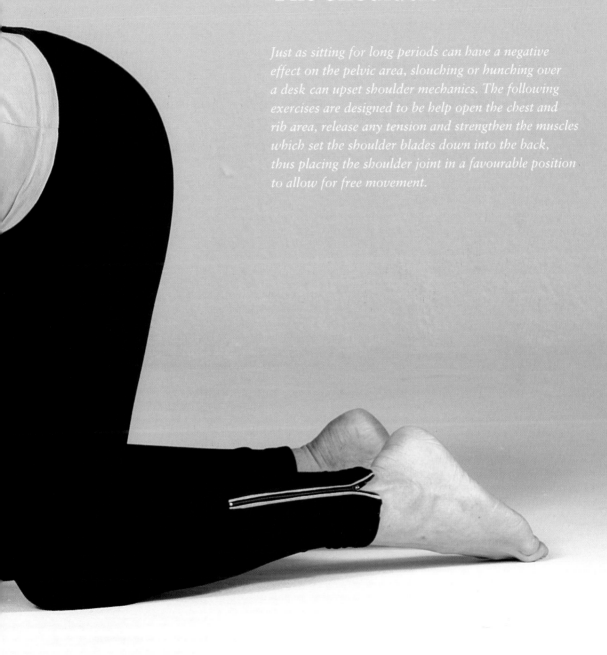

The Shoulders

Just as sitting for long periods can have a negative effect on the pelvic area, slouching or hunching over a desk can upset shoulder mechanics. The following exercises are designed to be help open the chest and rib area, release any tension and strengthen the muscles which set the shoulder blades down into the back, thus placing the shoulder joint in a favourable position to allow for free movement.

Dumb Waiter (*p*)

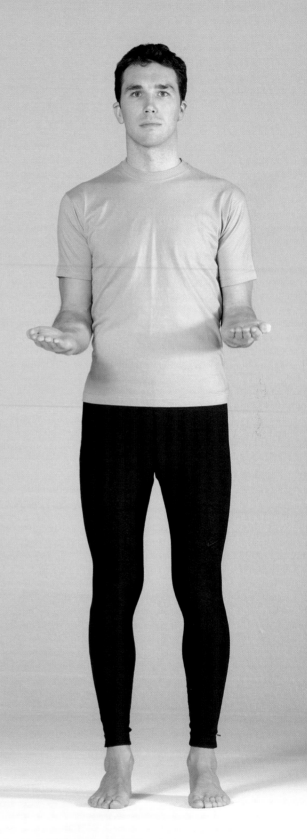

Aim

This is an ideal way to become aware of the shoulder blades and of their relationship with the ribcage. This exercise opens the chest, especially the front of the upper arms/shoulders (anterior deltoids) and strengthens the muscles between the shoulder blades (rhomboids).

Preparation

- Decide yourself if you want to sit on a chair or stand up for this exercise.
- If you choose to sit, position yourself well forward on a sturdy chair with your pelvis in neutral, feet planted on the floor hip-distance apart and your weight even on both buttocks.
- Alternatively, use the Standing Posture (see page 51) to give length to the entire body. Hold your arms, with your elbows tucked into your waist, palms facing upwards.

Action

1 Breathe in to prepare and lengthen up
  through the spine.
2 Breathe out, zip up and hollow.
3 Breathe in, still zipping.
4 Keeping your elbows in to your sides, take
  your hands backwards, opening them and
  working the muscles below the shoulder
  blades. Keep the shoulder blades down.
5 Breathe out and return the hands to the
  starting position.
6 Repeat five times.

Watchpoints

- Do not allow the upper back to arch as you
  take the arms back.
- If you find this very easy, check that your
  elbows are staying in and your shoulder
  blades are staying down.
- Keep the neck released.

Corkscrew (*p*)

Aim

This exercise teaches the correct placement and mechanics of the shoulders. It is called the corkscrew because the head lengthens up from the spine as the arms descend, like a cork popping out of a bottle.

Preparation

• Stand so the body is perfectly aligned as you did for the Standing Posture (see page 51).

Action

1 Breathe in wide and full to prepare and lengthen up through the spine.
2 As you breathe out, zip up and hollow (stay zipped throughout), then allow your arms to float up with the palms facing upwards.
3 Keep the upper shoulders relaxed and think of dropping the shoulder blades down towards the waist.
4 Clasp your hands lightly behind your head, breathe in and shrug your shoulders up to your ears. As you breathe out, lower them again.

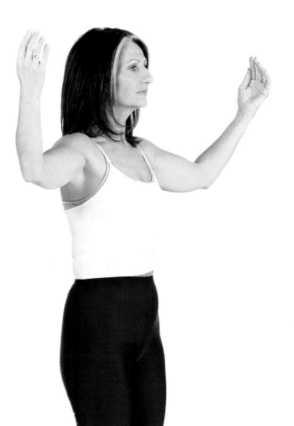

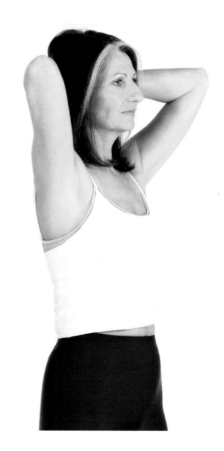

5 On the next inhalation, gently bring the elbows back a little without arching your back, so the shoulder blades come together.

6 Breathe out, release the shoulders and hands and bring them up, out and then down slowly to your side, opening them wide and engaging the muscles below the shoulder blades. As you do this, allow the head, neck and spine to lengthen up.

7 Repeat five times.

Watchpoints

- Keep your arms just a little in front of you as you raise and lower them, they should stay within your peripheral vision.
- Take care not to arch your back as you take your elbows back.

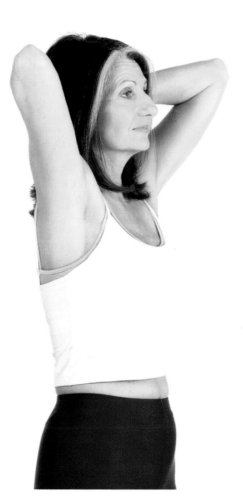

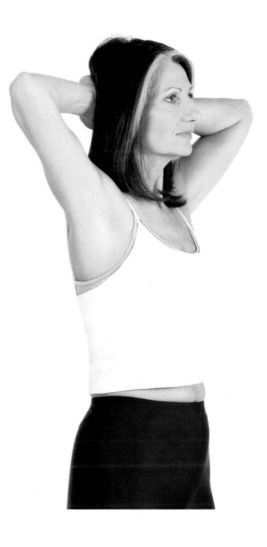

Threading a Needle (*p*)

Aim
Use this exercise to relax the upper back, especially the muscles around the shoulder girdle.

Preparation
- Come on to all fours with the hands under the shoulders and the knees under the hips.
- The neck should be long and the head in good alignment with the spine so you are looking straight down at the floor.

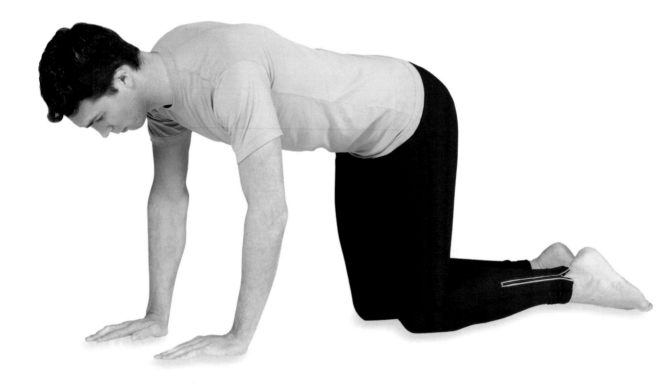

Action

1 Breathe in wide and full. Transfer your weight on to the left hand.

2 Breathe out, zip and hollow then lift your right hand up and return the back of the hand to the floor. The elbow should be open and relaxed.

3 Slide the right hand along the mat under the left arm, which bends. Keep both shoulders down into the back and relax the head.

4 Breathe in and relax in this position.

5 Breathe out and return to starting point, zipping and hollowing.

6 Repeat three times on each arm.

Watchpoint

• Only stretch as far as is comfortable.

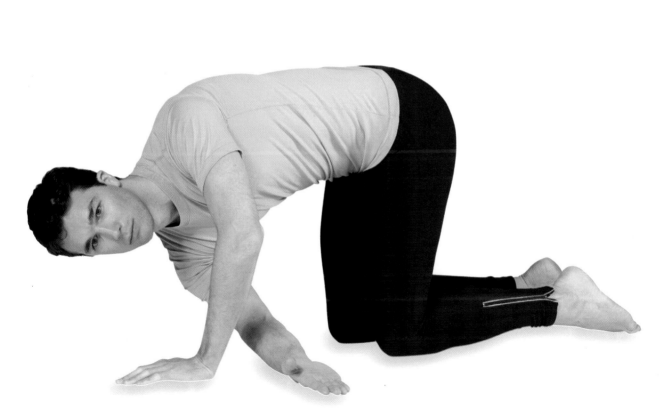

Eagle (y)

Aim
This exercise opens the chest and shoulders and separates the area between the shoulder blades.

Warning: those people with previously dislocated shoulders should proceed with caution.

Preparation
Get into the Standing Posture (see page 51).

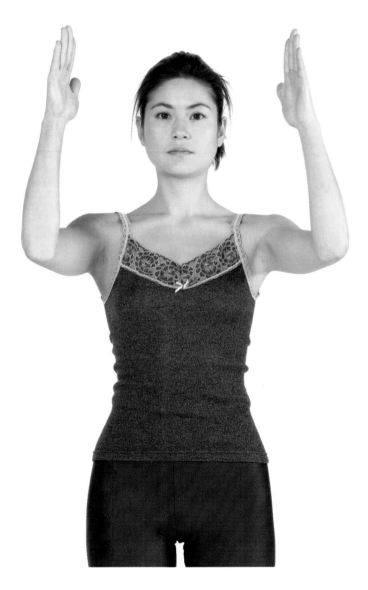

Action

1 Bring the right arm under the left, elbow bent and fingers toward the ceiling.
2 Twist the right hand so it comes around the left arm to the palm of the left hand.
3 Your arms should now be pointing straight up with your hands directly in your line of vision.
4 Repeat on the other side.

Watchpoints

- Don't let the arms or elbows drop too far – the hands should be in line with the forehead.
- Don't push the spine back through the shoulder blades – let them open and separate.

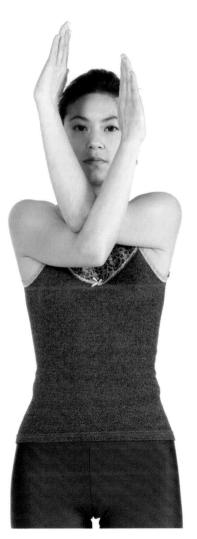

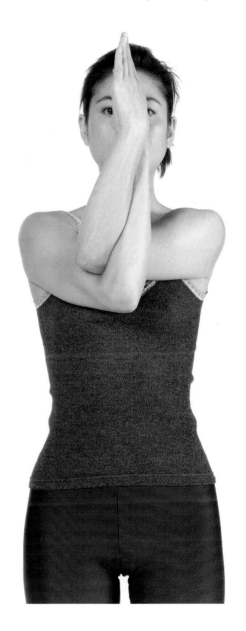

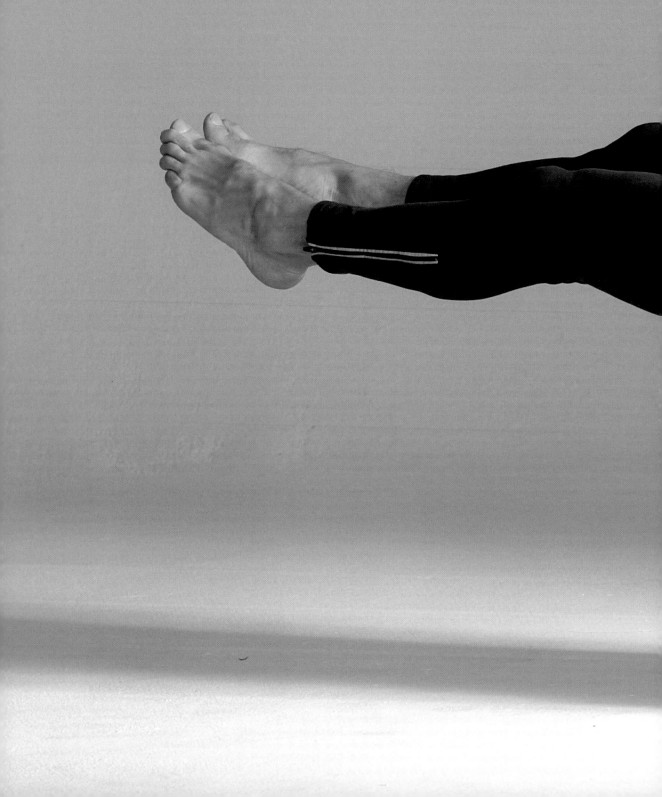

Inversions

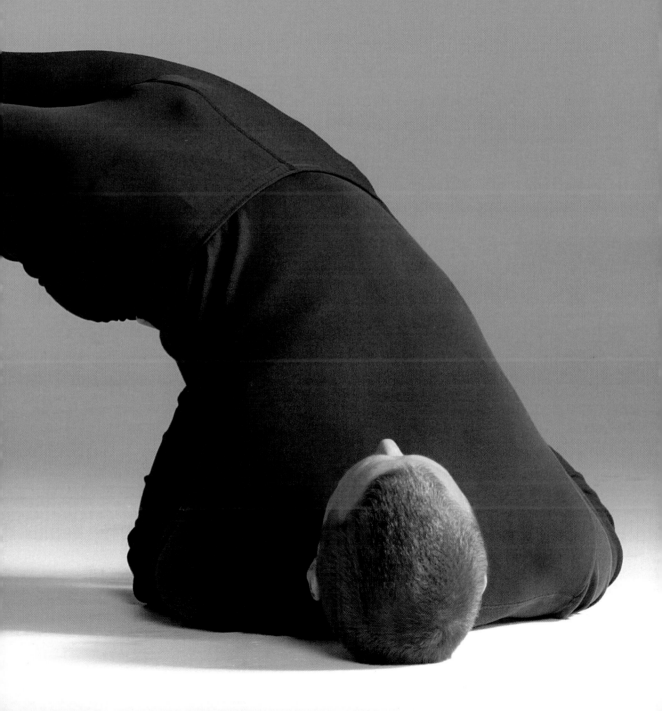

Legs Up the Wall (*p*)

This series of wall stretches looks deceptively easy. They require you to have your legs up a wall – a fabulous position for improving the circulation in the legs. Elevated, the 'calf pump' works doubly well. As the muscles tighten and relax, they help the veins to pump the blood back to the heart (venous return). If you suffer from varicose veins, which is where the valves in the veins have failed and blood is allowed to seep out into the surrounding tissue, there exists a blockage in the system, these exercises will help to clear the blockage.

The Starting Position

There is no elegant way to get into this position. The easiest way is to roll on to your side, shuffle your bottom up as close as you can to the wall and then swing your legs round and up. (On a practical note, you would be wise not to use a wall covered with your best designer wallpaper as you are likely to leave heel marks on it!) Move your buttocks as close to the wall as possible. If you have short hamstrings this will prove difficult so only come as close to the wall as is comfortable. Your tailbone should still touch the floor. Have the pelvis in neutral and put your head on a flat pillow if necessary.

NOTE: When you have finished the wall exercises roll on to your side and rest for a few minutes before standing up.

The Basic Wall Stretch

Aim

As well as relaxing and widening the torso, especially around the shoulder blades, this exercise will lengthen the entire spine.
It also improves the circulation in the legs.

Preparation

- Get into the Starting Position and, if you can, take your arms behind you soft and wide and relax them on to the floor. If not, leave them down by your sides.
- Remember to keep your ribcage calm – do not allow the upper back to arch – and allow the spine to lengthen and the neck to release.

Action

1 Work up to spending three minutes in this position. Bear in mind that if you are going to continue with the following exercises, you will be here for quite some time so judge it carefully.
2 When you have finished, gently bend the knees and bring your arms down by your sides.

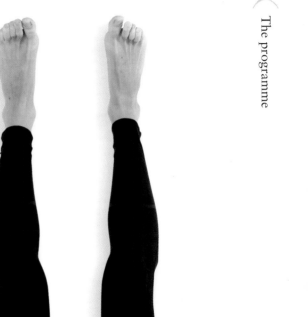

Ankle Circles

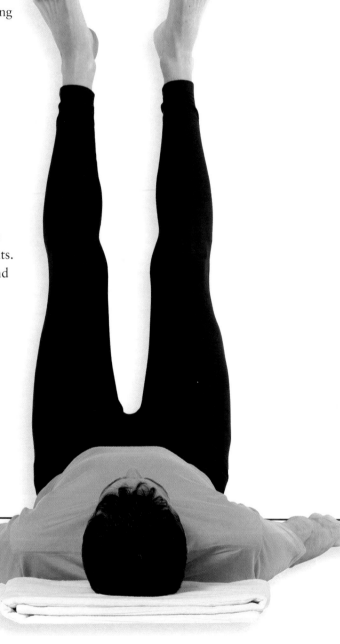

Aim

This exercise will stretch the hamstrings, work the muscles of the lower leg and mobilize and strengthen the ankle joints as well as improving circulation.

Preparation

- Get into position (see page 176).
- The legs should be hip-distance apart and parallel.
- Check that you are square to the wall and not at an angle and that your pelvis is in neutral.

Action

1 Keeping the legs completely still, rotate the feet outwardly, circling from the ankle joints. You should be circling very, very slowly and as far as you can.
2 Repeat 10 circles in each direction.

Watchpoints

- Don't just twiddle the toes around, work from the ankle joints.
- When it says keep the legs still, that means still! And parallel.

Point and Flex

Aim

You'll feel this one in your shins. It works all the muscles of the foot and lower leg and stretches the hamstrings.

Preparation

- As for Ankle Circles.

Action

1 Keep the legs parallel and hip-distance apart and point your toes up towards the ceiling.
2 Flex the toes down towards your face.
3 Keeping the toes flexed, flex the feet towards your face, lengthening through the heels.
4 Relax the toes.
5 Repeat 10 times.

Watchpoints

- Make sure that your tailbone is still in contact with the floor.
- Bend your knees a little if the stretch in your hamstrings is too great.

The programme

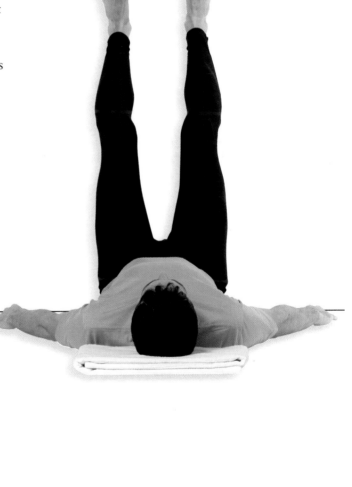

Downward Facing Dog (*y*)

Aim

Most of the body is used in this dynamic posture, making it a great toning exercise. It elongates the spine and releases tension in the entire spinal column as well as strengthening the arms, wrists and shoulders and opening up the backs of the legs and the hips. The exercise is a very complex one, so break it into sections and concentrate on getting each bit right. It's better to repeat the exercise a few times than only do it once incorrectly.

Warning: avoid this exercise if you have high blood pressure, carpal tunnel syndrome or glaucoma, or any wrist, disc or retinal injuries.

Preparation

• Begin in the Resting Child position, explained on page 118.

Action

1 Extend the arms in front of you, shoulder-distance apart with the palms extended and the fingers facing forwards. The elbows should be off the floor.
2 As you breathe out, come on to all fours with the hips above the knees.
3 Release tension in the hips by allowing them to sway gently from side to side.
4 Tuck the toes under the heels.
5 Breathing out, very gently let the hips move up towards the ceiling.
6 Your foundation should be in the balls of the feet and the open palms of the hands.
7 Relax the ankles to let the heel drop and open out the back of the leg.
8 Release the thighs and knees slightly to let the hips float in relationship to the feet. There should be a similar connection to that of the standing alignment, except the centre of gravity has changed quite severely.
9 Breathe out following the abdominals back towards the spine (see yoga breathing on page 33). Soften and release the area at the back of the hips and lengthen the back of the waist.
10 Soften between the shoulder blades and allow the arms to move back towards the shoulders without bending or collapsing them. This will lengthen the spine and the back of the neck and open out the area between the shoulders.
11 Transfer the weight back slightly into the heel.
12 Bend the knees to the floor and go into the Resting Child position.

 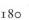

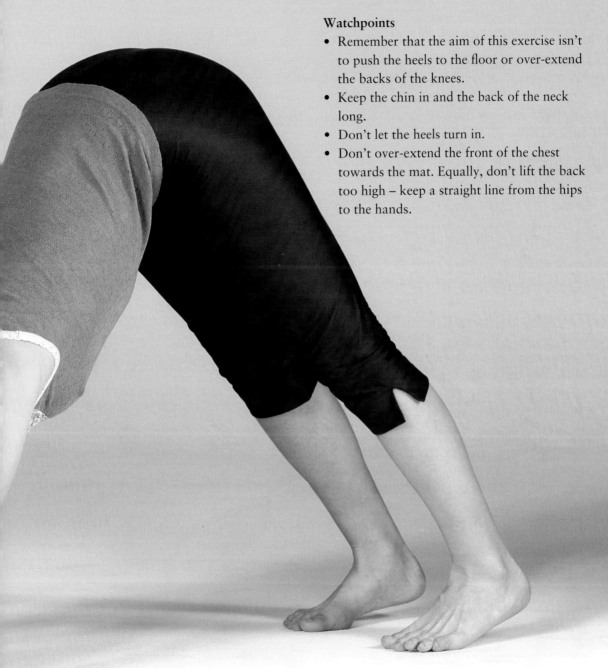

Watchpoints

- Remember that the aim of this exercise isn't to push the heels to the floor or over-extend the backs of the knees.
- Keep the chin in and the back of the neck long.
- Don't let the heels turn in.
- Don't over-extend the front of the chest towards the mat. Equally, don't lift the back too high – keep a straight line from the hips to the hands.

Shoulder Stand Against a Wall (*y*)

Aim

This is a simpler version of a shoulder stand, but is still an intermediate level exercise that improves circulation and reduces fluid retention in the legs, ankles and feet. Included is the simplest version – use this if you find the others difficult or if you are menstruating.

Warning: this exercise is not advisable if you have a weak heart, a detached retina, neck injuries or if you are menstruating. Be careful if you have high blood pressure.

Equipment

A blanket (optional).

Preparation

- Place the mat with one end against the wall.
- Get into the Starting Position described for Legs Up the Wall on page 176.

Action

1 Bend the knees, keeping the feet hip-distance apart.
2 Very slowly, tuck the tailbone under to roll up the spine.
3 As the spine comes up, start walking the feet up the wall so that they are at right angles to the knees.
4 Support the middle of the back with the hands, elbows on the mat.
5 Tuck the tailbone under and open out the front of the hips.
6 When you are ready, release the hands and very gently roll down vertebra by vertebra on to the mat. Bend the knees to your chest and carefully roll on to your side. From here, slowly come up to sitting.

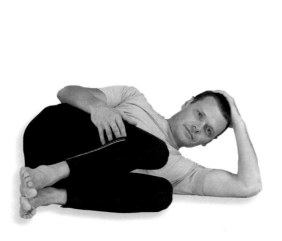
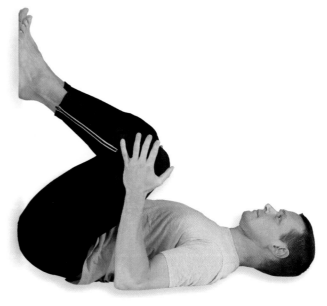

Simple Variation

Watchpoints

- Remember that the lift in the body comes from lengthening the spine.
- If the back of the neck is tight, place a blanket under the shoulders to allow more freedom (see Watchpoints page 185)

Prepare the same way, but as you bring your legs up the wall, keep them pointing straight up towards the ceiling, with the feet flexed. Bring the arms out to the sides and let them rest palm facing up, wherever comfortable. If you want, take the legs out into a wide V-shape.

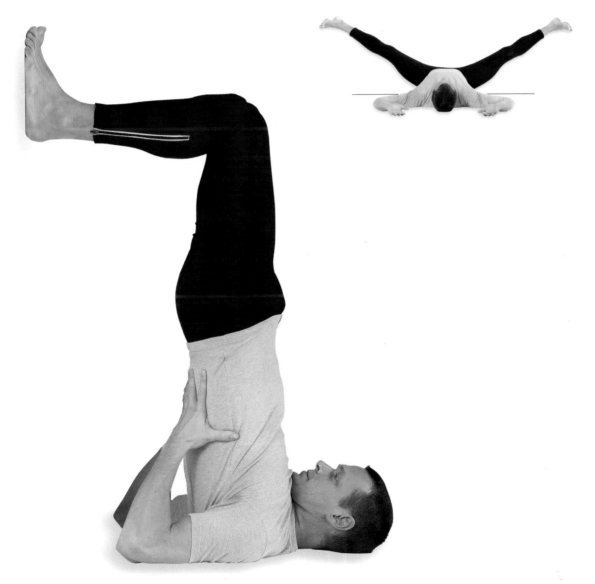

Shoulder Stand (*y*) (*advanced*)

Aim

This wonderful exercise has many benefits. Use it to relieve mental and physical fatigue as well as improve the function of the metabolic, digestive, nervous, glandular and reproductive systems. It also increases blood flow to the brain, stimulates the thyroid gland, sedates and neutralizes the nervous system while improving circulation and reducing fluid retention in the legs, ankles and feet. Further benefits include toning internal organs – especially the reproductive organs – and promoting healthy bowel function.

Warning: this exercise is not advisable if you have a weak heart, a detached retina, neck injuries or if you are menstruating. Be careful if you have high blood pressure.

Equipment

A blanket (optional).

Preparation

• Sit with your legs stretched out in front of you.

Action

1 Before going into an inverted posture, get a sense of length in the spine. Place the hands behind the hips, fingertips pointing backwards. Drop the shoulder blades down, open out the front of the chest, tuck in the chin and allow the spine to be long, creating space between the ribcage and the hips.
2 Very gently, roll back on the mat, the arms come down by your side with palms face down. Raise the knees as you roll backwards.

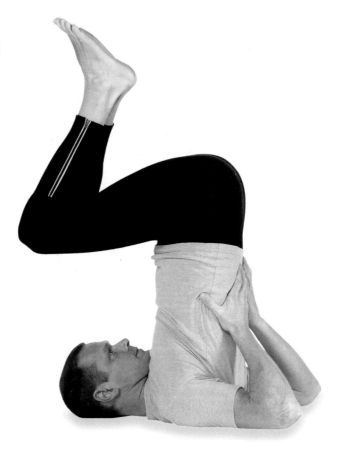

3 Push down with the palms of the hands to help bring the knees on to your forehead. Place the hands on to the middle of the back for support, with the elbows firmly planted on the mat.

4 Bring the elbows together and slide the hands down the back towards the mat. Find your foundation in the shoulders and the backs of the upper arms.

5 Lift the hips to create length in the spine. The hips move away from the ribcage, in the same way as for a Standing Posture, only upside down.

6 From here, straighten one leg up at a time.

7 Stay in this position for as long as you are comfortable then rest the knees down towards the forehead. Release the hand back on to the mat palms facing down then roll back on to the mat, lengthening the spine vertebra by vertebra.

Watchpoints

• The important thing to remember is that the lift in the body comes from lengthening the spine. Lift from the hips, not from the feet.

• If the back of the neck is tight, place a blanket under the shoulders and have the head resting on the floor to allow more freedom.

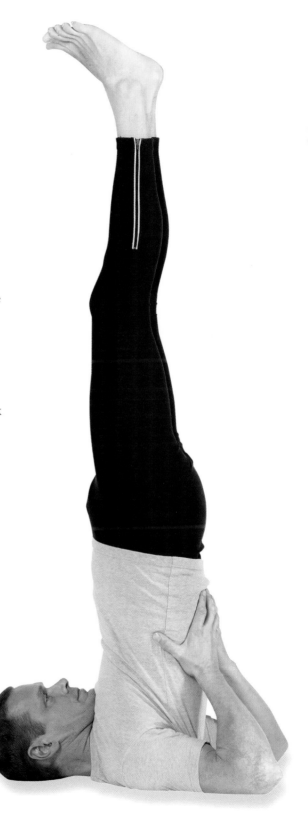

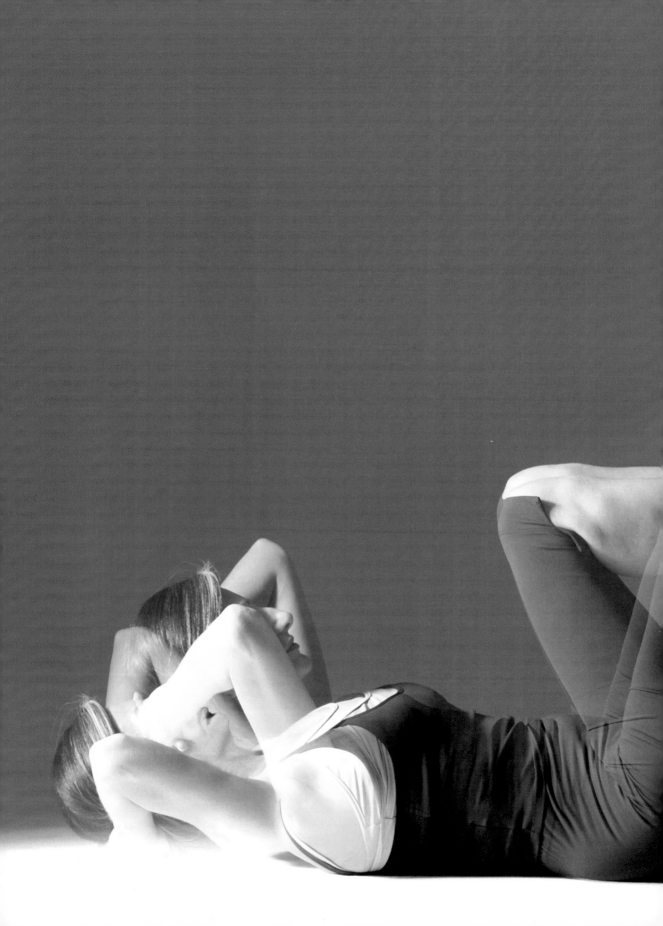

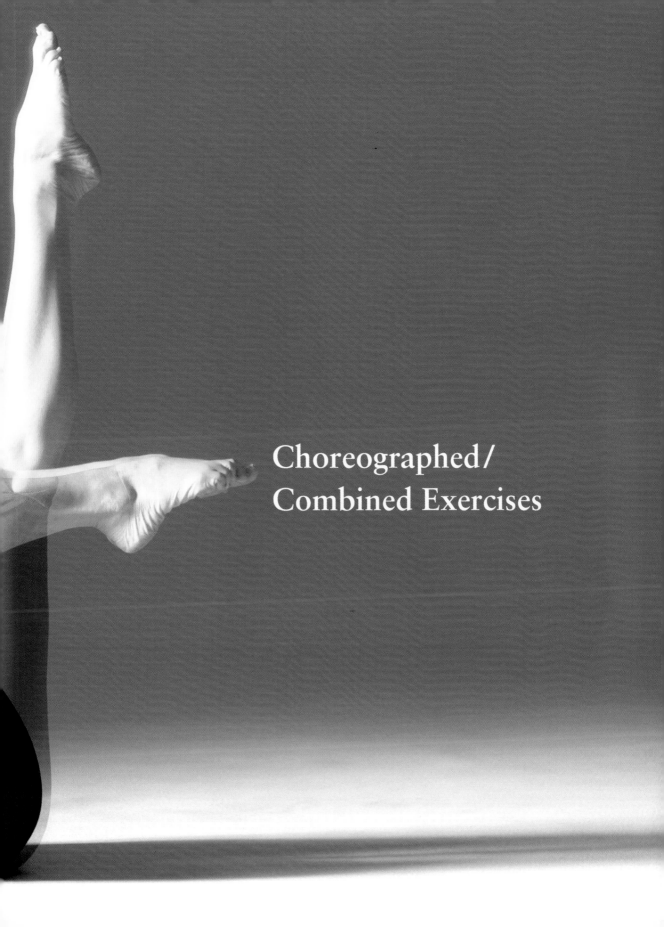

Choreographed/
Combined Exercises

Starbugs (p)

Aim

These co-ordination exercises incorporate all the skills you have learned for your Pilates exercises.

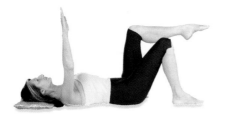

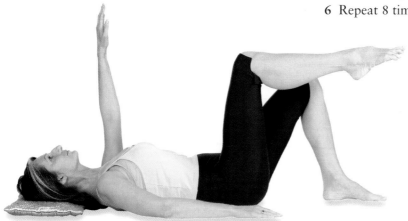

Preparation

- Lie in the Relaxation Position (see page 48).

Action

1 Breathe in wide and full to prepare.
2 Breathe out, zip up and hollow (stay zipped now), and fold your right knee up towards your chest to a 90° angle, at the same time raising your left arm to vertical.
3 Breathe in wide and full.
4 Breathe out and lower your foot and arm back to the floor.
5 Repeat this movement with the opposite arm and leg.
6 Repeat 8 times with each arm and leg.

Watchpoints

- Although you are working the opposite arm and leg it helps to imagine that they are connected with a piece of string, like a puppet.
- Try to keep the action natural and flowing.
- Remember everything you have learnt about good upper-body movement: your neck is released, your ribcage is calm, your shoulder blades are down into the back.
- Keep the pelvis still and in neutral – lower abdominals stay hollow.

Intermediate

Preparation
- Lie in the Relaxation Position (see page 48).

Action
1 Breathe in wide and full to prepare.
2 Breathe out, zip up and hollow (stay zipped now), and fold your left knee up towards your chest to a 90° angle, at the same time, raising both arms directly above your shoulders, palms facing away from you.
3 Breathe in and check that your pelvis is still in neutral and your shoulder blades are down into your back so that your upper body is open.
4 Breathe out, and take your arms in a backstroke movement as if to touch the floor (do not force them).
5 At the same time, extend the leg away from you at a 45° angle. You should still be zipped.
6 Breathe in, fold the knee in and lift the arms directly above the shoulders.
7 Breathe out and return the foot and arms to the floor.
8 Repeat 5 times on each side.

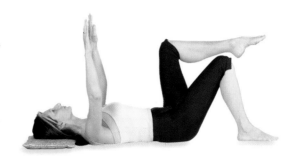

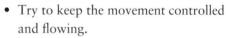

Watchpoints
- As you take your arms behind you keep your breastbone soft and your ribcage down – do not let it flare.
- Your pelvis must stay quite still and stable as the leg both folds in and extends away.
- The lower abdominals should stay zipped throughout.
- Try to keep the movement controlled and flowing.

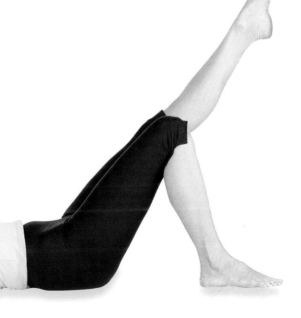

Advanced

This requires strong abdominals and excellent core stability.

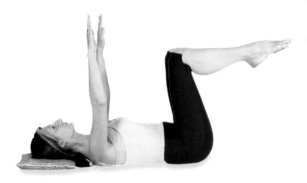

Preparation
- Lie in the Relaxation Position (see page 48). Slowly zip up and hollow and bring your knees up to your chest one at a time.
- Stay in neutral.
- Have your arms directly above your shoulders, palms facing away from you.
- Your shoulder blades should remain down, your upper body is soft and open.

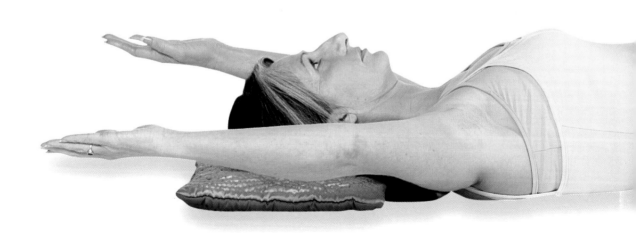

Action

1 Breathe in wide and full to prepare.
2 Breathe out, zip up and hollow (stay zipped throughout).
3 Take your arms behind you and touch the floor if you can (do not force them).
4 At the same time, extend one leg away from you at an angle of above 45° to the floor.
5 Breathe and return to the starting position, that is, knees folded and arms above the shoulders.
6 Repeat 8 times to each side.

Watchpoints

- As for other Starbugs – use your centre and stay neutral!
- Do not allow the back to arch.

Single Leg Stretch (*p*)

Aim

This is a classical Pilates exercise best taught in
simple stages. It challenges both the abdominal
muscles and your co-ordination – in fact it
combines *all* the eight principles.

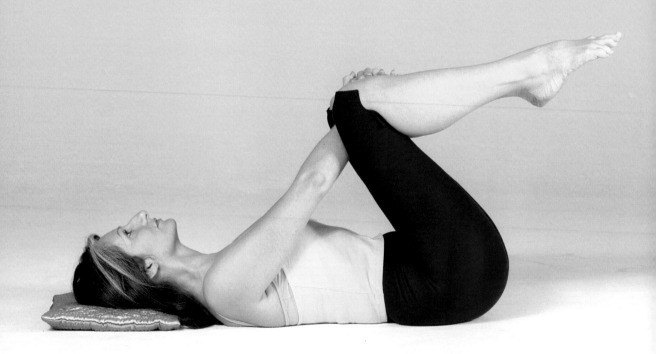

Stage One

Preparation
• Lie in the Relaxation Position (see page 48).

Action
1 Breathe in wide and full to prepare.
2 Breathe out, zip up and hollow, then fold one knee at a time to your chest.
3 Breathe in and hold your left knee with both hands. Keep your neck released, your elbows open and your breastbone soft with the shoulder blades sliding down into your back.
4 Breathe out, zip up and hollow (stay zipped throughout), then slowly straighten the right leg up into the air. Keep your back anchored into the floor.
5 Breathe in and bend the knee back in. Change legs.
6 Repeat ten times with each leg. Keep control of your legs; do not allow them to fall away from you – your back must stay anchored to the floor.

When this becomes easy – and only when – you may try the more advanced Stage Two.

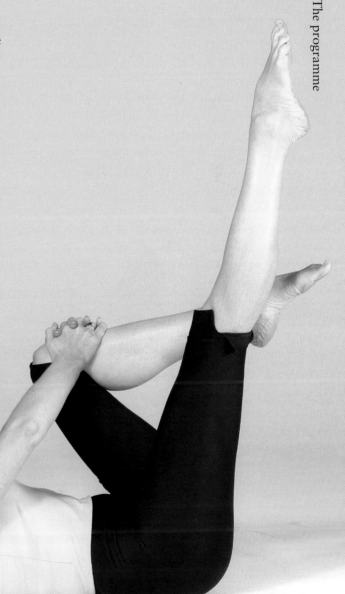

Stage Two

Preparation
- Lie in the Relaxation Position (see page 48)

Action

1 Breathe in to prepare.
2 Breathe out, zip up and hollow, then fold your knees up to your chest one at a time. The toes should be just touching, but not the heels. Keep your feet softly pointed.
3 Place your hands on the outside of your calves. Breathe in, check that your elbows are open to enable the chest to expand fully. Your shoulder blades are down into your back.
4 Breathe out, zip up and hollow (stay zipped throughout), soften your breastbone and curl the upper body off the floor.
5 Breathe in and place the right hand on the outside of the right ankle and the left hand on the inside of the right knee.
6 Breathe out and slowly stretch your left leg away so that it is at right angles to the floor. The toes are softly pointed.
7 Breathe in wide and full, as you begin to bend the leg back to your chest, bringing it back into your shoulder.
8 Change hands so that your left hand is on the outside of your left leg and your right hand on the inside of your left knee.

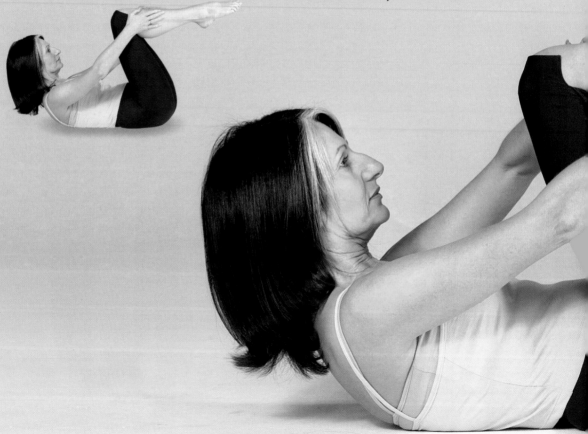

9 Breathe out still zipping up and hollowing, and stretch the right leg away so that it is at right angles to the floor. Do not take it too close to the floor.

10 Breathe in as the leg returns.

11 Repeat ten stretches with each leg, making sure that you have a strong centre throughout and that your shoulder blades stay down into your back and your elbows are open.

Watchpoints

- Keep zipping and hollowing throughout and do not allow the back to arch, but ensure the pelvis stays neutral.
- Keep your neck released and the upper body open, shoulder blades down.
- Make sure you keep the length on both sides of your waist – do not allow one side to shorten.

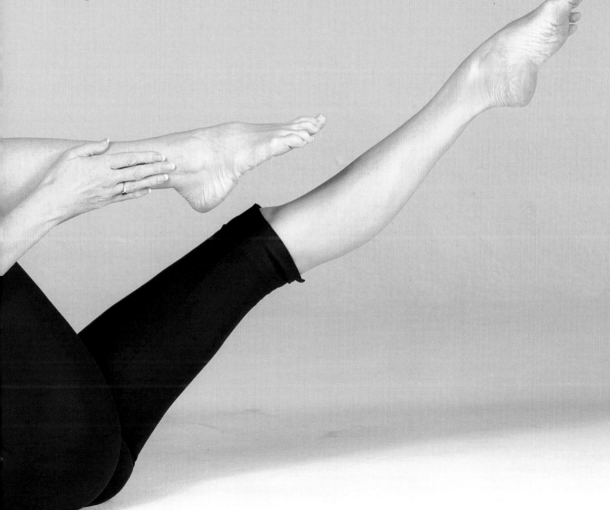

Arm Openings (*p*)

Aim

This has to be the most relaxing, feel-good exercise in the Pilates programme. If you stay completely aware of your arm and hand as it displaces the air moving through space, you will achieve a sense of openness while stabilizing and centring. This exercise will also open the upper body and stretch the pectoral muscles, while gently and safely rotating the spine.

Warning: as this exercise involves rotation of the spine, take advice if you have a disc-related injury.

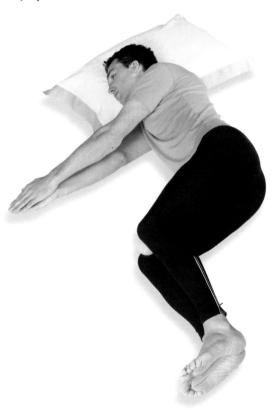

Equipment

A plump pillow, and a tennis ball (optional).

Preparation

- Lie on your side with your head on a pillow and your knees curled up at right angles to your body. Your back should be in a straight line, but with its natural curve.
- Place a tennis ball between your knees (the idea is for the tennis ball to keep your knees and pelvis in good alignment).
- Align all your bones – feet, ankles, knees, hips and shoulders – and extend your arms in front of you, with your palms together, at shoulder height.

Action

1 Breathe in to prepare and lengthen through the spine.
2 Breathe out and zip up and hollow. Stay zipped and hollowed throughout.
3 Breathe in and slowly open the top arm in an arc so that your upper body rotates. Keep the elbow soft. Keep your eyes on your hand so that the head follows the arm movement. You are aiming to touch the floor behind you, but do not force the arm past the line of the shoulder joint.
4 Try to keep your knees together and your pelvis still.
5 Breathe out as you bring the arm back in an arc to rest on the other hand again.
6 Repeat five times, then curl up on the other side and repeat.

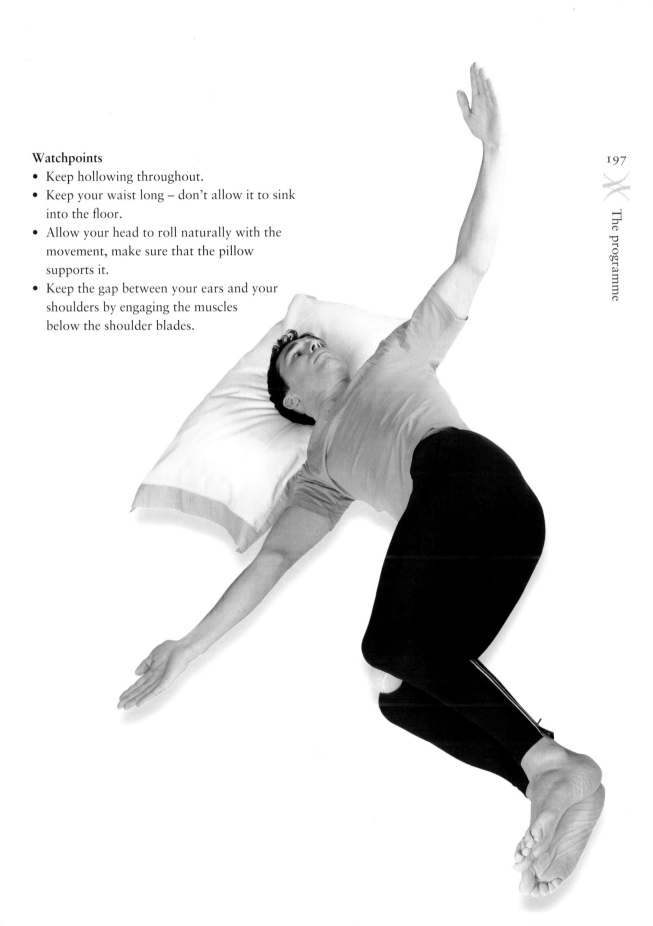

Watchpoints

- Keep hollowing throughout.
- Keep your waist long – don't allow it to sink into the floor.
- Allow your head to roll naturally with the movement, make sure that the pillow supports it.
- Keep the gap between your ears and your shoulders by engaging the muscles below the shoulder blades.

Cat and Dog (*y*)

Aim

The Cat posture opens up the back and spine, making it a great way to prepare for the Cobra, a Sun Salutation or any demanding backbend. It's also good for menstrual problems and bringing blood to the spine.

Warning: avoid this exercise if you have disc problems.

Preparation

- Start on all fours with your hands under the shoulders, your feet under the hips and your legs parallel.
- Gently tuck in the chin and look down between the hands.
- Lengthen out between the ribs and the hips and ensure the spine is in a neutral position (explained in Finding Neutral on page 49).
- As you breathe out, feel the abdomen scoop and hollow as the deep abdominal muscles are engaged.

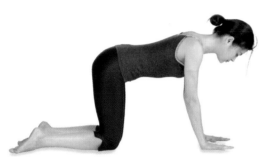

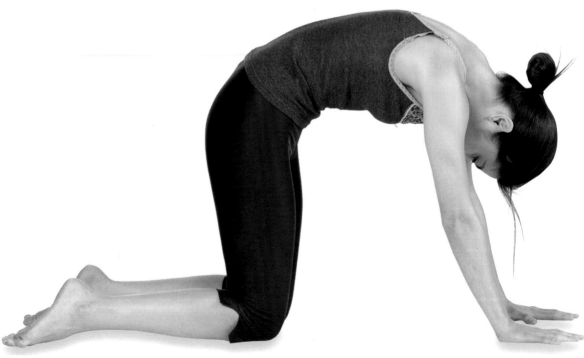

Action

1 Tuck the tailbone under the hips to allow the back of the waist to open out. Relax the front of the hips and move them from side to side, releasing any tension. Come back to neutral.

2 Drop the abdomen down towards the mat, keeping length in the spine. The abdomen will scoop back on the exhalation and the deep abdominals will be activated.

3 Come back to neutral.

4 Using very small movements from the area of the lower back, move up and down. Although you are moving the lower back, the movement is actually coming from the tailbone and hips.

5 Release the hips, allowing the movement to become more fluid. As it does so, gradually extend your awareness along the spine to the middle back and up through the shoulders and finally to the back of the neck and the head.

6 Once the entire length of the spine is being used, slowly decrease the amount of movement and come back to neutral.

Watchpoints

- Don't rush each movement; keep them free, flowing and connected all the way along the spine.
- Breathe in as the head comes up; breathe out as the head goes down.
- Make sure the hands are under the shoulders and the knees are under the hips.
- Start off with small movements backwards and forwards then increase the movement along the spine once it has become fluid.
- Keep the movement from the back of the waist, not between the shoulder blades.

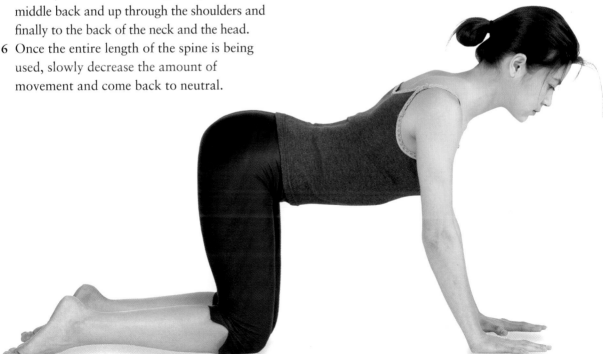

Sun Salutation (y)

Aim

This flowing sequence, called a Sun Salutation or suryanamaskar, is based on the ancient practice of worshipping the sun. It combines many of the exercises already described in this book, but to achieve a sense of flow don't cut corners or forget the details that you've already learnt. This is a great way to condition the whole body, developing strength, flexibility, flow and co-ordination. It lubricates the joints and warms up the muscles, improves circulation, reduces lethargy and can help combat depression.

Warning: if you have ME you should be careful.

Preparation

- Begin in the Standing Posture (see page 51). with your feet at the front of the mat.
- Don't worry about the breath at first, but once you've started to become familiar with the sequence, introduce it to help you get a greater sense of flow. It's fairly straightforward: breathe in when you open up and out when you close down the body. At one point, you will also be instructed to hold the breath for a short time.

Action

1 As you breath out, let your arms float up to the sides.
2 Turn the palms up towards the ceiling bringing the hands above the head, shoulder-distance apart. Keep the shoulders soft.
3 As you breath out, bring the hands out to the side and come down into a forward bend.
4 Place both hands on the mat and bring the fingertips in line with the toes. Don't worry if you have to bend your knees.

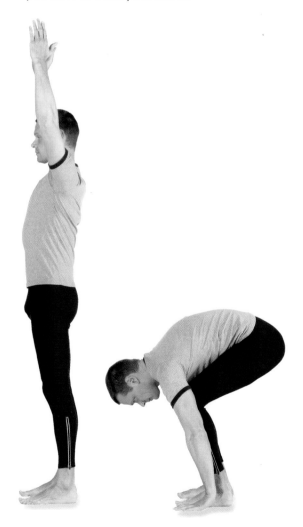

5 Breathing in, extend the right foot backwards and drop the right knee on to the mat. Make sure the left heel is under the left knee and release the hips.

6 Hold the breath, lift the right knee and, keeping the hips where they are, sweep the left foot back alongside the right. You are now in a straight line from the shoulders to the heels.

7 Drop the knees to the floor and arch the back down towards the floor.

8 Breathing out, take the chest straight down between the hands with the elbows bent close to your sides.

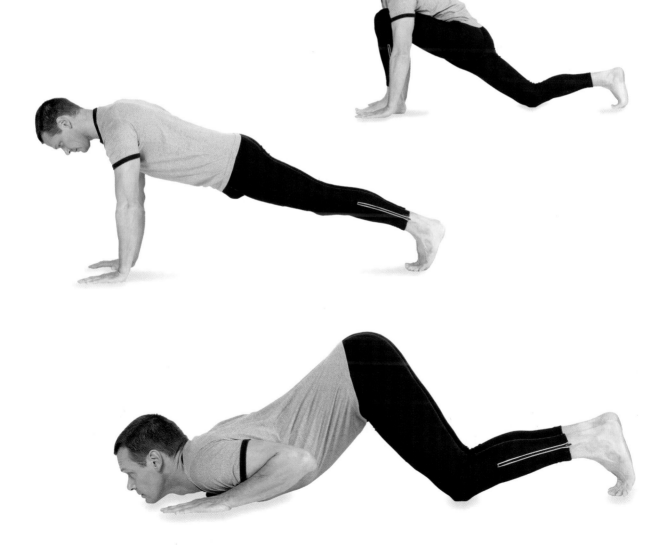

9 Breathe in, extending forward as you move up into the Full Cobra (see page 112). Keep the chin tucked in and the shoulders away from the ears.

10 On an exhalation, tuck the toes under the heels and push back into a Downward Facing Dog (see page 180).

11 On an inhalation, move the right foot forward between the hands, keeping the fingertips and toes in line. Rest the left knee on the mat.

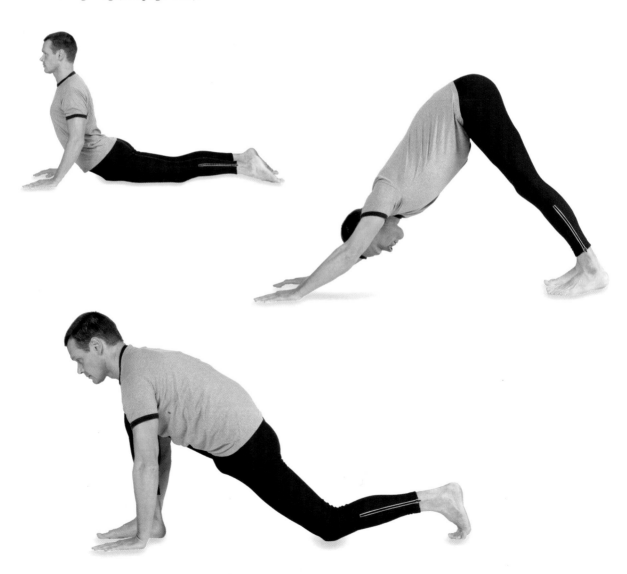

12 As you breathe out, lift the left knee and push off with the left foot, bringing it alongside the right into a forward bend.

13 Floating the arms out to the side, breathe in and come up, with a flat back, by dropping the tailbone down and bringing the hands above the head with the shoulders relaxed.

14 Repeat, starting by extending the left foot back this time.

Watchpoints

• Try not to let the momentum of the exercise push you further into each position, let it flow easily.

• Get a sense of flow by keeping the movements smooth.

• Introduce the breath once you become familiar with the sequence.

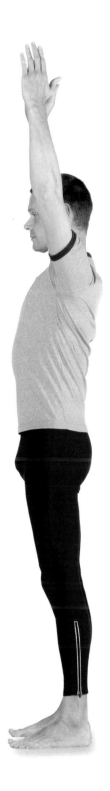

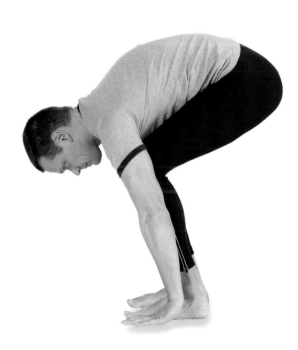

Rolling Down Cobra (*y*)

Aim

Move into this more advanced position for a deeper, more effective opening of the spine, abdomen and back muscles. It will also invigorate the heart and lungs, stimulate and massage the abdominal organs and regenerate the muscles of the torso.

Warning: avoid this exercise if you have any spinal problems.

Preparation

- Start on all fours with the hands slightly in front of the shoulders, the feet hip-distance apart and the legs parallel.
- Lengthen out between the ribs and the hips and ensure the spine is in a neutral position (explained in Finding Neutral see page 49).

Action

1 Take the hands forwards, about 30 centimetres, and tuck the tailbone under to open out the back of the waist. When going into a backward bend, it's important to keep the spine long by moving the tailbone away from the back of the head. Tuck the tailbone under the hips, so the spine is in a forward arch.

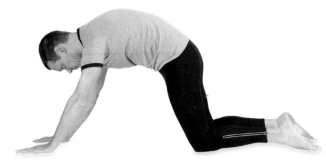

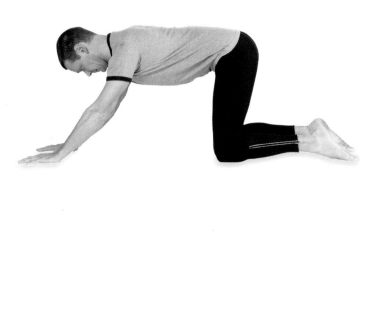

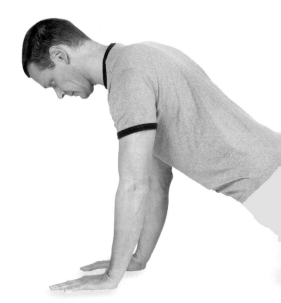

2 Start to take the hips forward and down to the floor moving the spine from a forward arch into a back arch, leading with the tailbone.

3 For the moment, keep the arms straight. This allows the ribcage to be lifted and the lower back to be lengthened as the hips and ribcage separate.

4 The head comes up as a result of the movement along the length of the spine. Keep the buttocks soft.

5 At the top of the movement, drop the shoulders towards the waist and let the elbows bend.

6 Repeat a few times without holding for too long at the top of the movement. Come back into the starting position between each repetition.

7 When you have finished, come into the Resting Child position (see page 118).

Watchpoints

- Be aware that you are moving from a forward arch into a backbend.
- Keep the tailbone tucked right under the hips for as long as possible.
- Roll along the spine like a wave, from the tailbone to the back of the head.
- Don't drop the head back at the top of the move.
- Keep the back of the neck long, with the eyes looking towards the horizon.

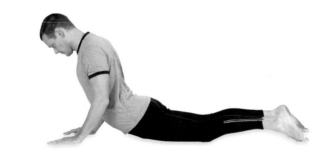

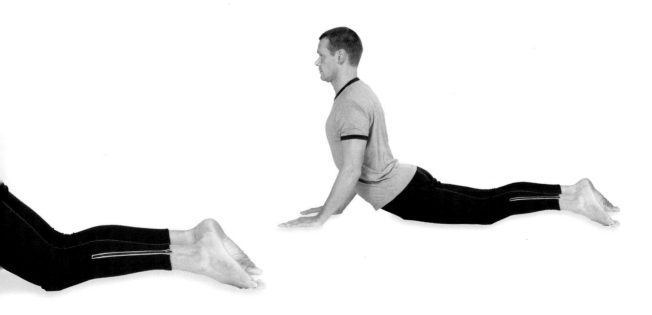

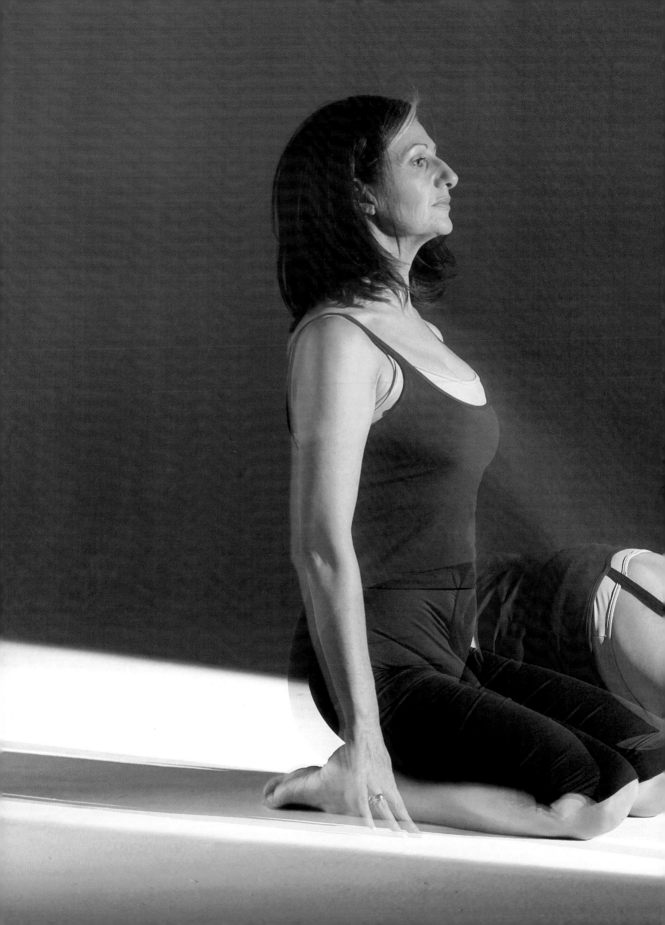

Relaxation

A Short Relaxation (*p*)

Aim

Use this technique to recognize and release tension from the body – it's the perfect way to end the day or any of your workout sessions. Ideally, you should persuade a friend to read the instructions to you, otherwise try taping them.

Equipment

A large pillow (optional).

Preparation

- Lie in the Relaxation Position (see page 48) and allow your whole body to melt down into the floor, lengthening and widening.
- Place a large pillow under your knees, if you want.

Action

1 Take your awareness down to your feet and soften the soles, uncurling the toes.
2 Soften your ankles.
3 Soften your calves.
4 Release your knees.
5 Release your thighs.
6 Allow your hips to open.
7 Allow the small of your back to sink into the floor as though you are sinking down into the folds of a hammock.
8 Feel the length of your spine.
9 Take your awareness down to your hands, stretch your fingers away from your palms, feel the centre of your palms opening.
10 Then allow the fingers to curl and the palms to soften.

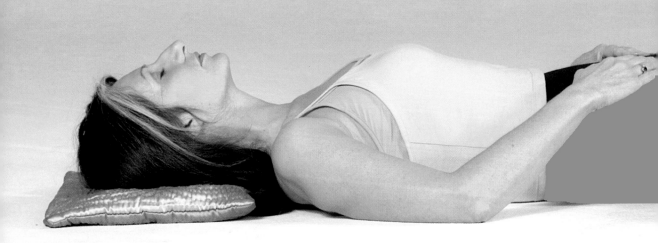

11 Allow your elbows to open.

12 Allow the front of your shoulders to soften.

13 With each out breath allow your shoulder blades to widen.

14 Allow your breastbone to soften.

15 Allow your neck to release.

16 Check your jaw, it should be loose and free.

17 Allow your tongue to widen at its base and rest comfortably at the bottom of your mouth.

18 Your lips are softly closed.

19 Your eyes are softly closed.

20 Your forehead is wide and smooth and completely free of lines.

21 Your face feels soft.

22 Your body feels soft and warm.

23 Your spine is gently released down into the floor.

24 Observe your breathing, but do not interrupt it. Simply enjoy its natural rhythm.

To Come Out of the Relaxation:
Very gently allow your head to roll to one side, allowing its own weight to move it. Slowly roll it back to the centre and then allow it to roll to the other side. Bring it back to the centre. Wriggle your fingers . . . and then your toes. Very slowly roll on to one side and rest there for a few minutes before slowly getting up.

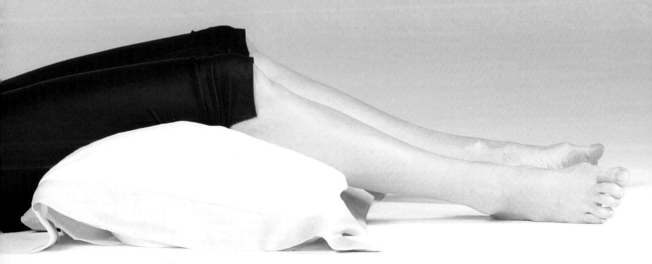

Seated Relaxation (*y*)

Aim

This technique is a wonderful way to open
the hips and help to strengthen the core postural
muscles. It allows the nervous system to
integrate the adjustments made to the body
during exercise and calms the mind.

Equipment

A plump pillow.

Preparation

- Come into a comfortable, cross-legged
  position.
- Lean forward lightly and wedge the pillow
  under the back of the hips (this stops them
  from rolling back, giving support and
  allowing the muscles in the groin to release).
- Use your sitting bones for alignment and to
  find your foundation.

Action

1 Bring your weight forward slightly to relieve
  the pressure in your back then very gently
  transfer your weight backwards again,
  allowing the spine to stack up vertebra by
  vertebra until it is in a vertical position.
2 For the moment, rest your hands on your
  feet.
3 Allow the shoulder blades to soften and the
  front of the chest to open. Keep the spine
  long and the chin tucked in gently.
4 Place your hands on your knees, either facing
  down or facing up with the thumb and index
  finger touching and the other fingers open
  and long. Alternatively, lay your hands in
  your lap, one inside the other.
5 As you breathe in, let the breath move into
  the top of the chest.
6 As you breathe out, follow the breath into
  the bodydown, past the abdomen and
  tailbone. Allow the breath to taper off.
7 Wait for the inhalation. Let it move towards
  you.
8 Breathe in and allow the breath to fill the
  chest once more.
9 Stay in this position as long as you like
  and continue to follow the movement of
  the breath. If at any point you start to feel
  a strain in the back, continue the relaxation
  lying on your back.

Simple Variation

Sit in a comfortable cross-legged position with your back against a wall and your hips tight in against the skirting board. Allow the back to be supported and follow the breath as directed above.

Watchpoint

- You shouldn't be sitting on the cushion, just using it to support the back of the hips.

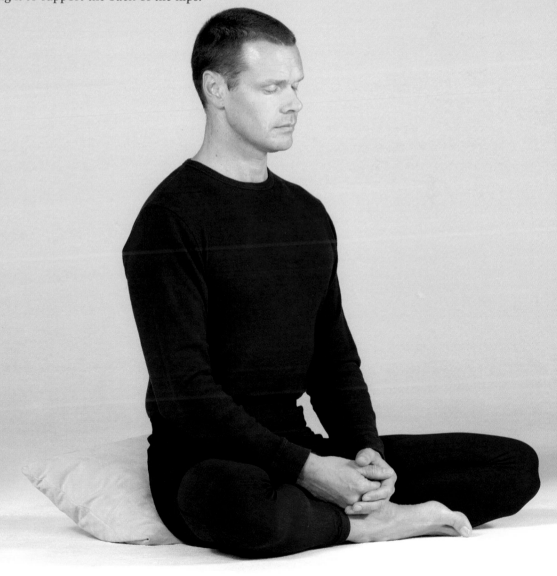

7 Workouts One

We have suggested seven workouts for you to try. Each is perfectly balanced and should take around 20–30 minutes to complete. Some of the exercises have different levels of difficulty. Please work at the right level for you.

Beach Ball Hamstring Stretch (*p*)	p. 86	
Forward Bend (*y*)	p. 94	
Simple Standing Side Reach (*p*)	p. 138	
Standing Spinal Twist (*y*)	p. 130	
Dumb Waiter (*p*)	p. 166	
Neck Rolls (*p*)	p. 70	
Pelvic Stability – Knee Turn Out (*p*)	p. 63	
Curl Up (*p*)	p. 88	
Single Leg Stretch – Stage One or Two (*p*)	p. 192	
Bridge (*y*)	p. 116	
Basic Wall Stretch (*p*)	p. 177	
Ankle Circles (*p*)	p. 178	
Diamond Press (*p*)	p. 102	
Downward Facing Dog (*y*)	p. 180	
Resting Child (*p+y*)	p. 118	

Two

Starfish (*p*)	p. 68	
Bridge (*y*)	p. 116	
Hip Flexor Stretch (*p*)	p. 156	
Hip Rolls (*p*)	p. 122	
Seated Side Bend (*y*)	p. 145	
Eagle (*y*)	p. 172	
Corkscrew (*p*)	p. 168	
Cobbler (*y*)	p. 158	
The Hundred (*p*)	p. 90	
Extended Cobra (*y*)	p. 110	
Cat and Dog (*y*)	p. 198	
Resting Child (*p+y*)	p. 118	

Three

Neck Rolls (*p*)	p. 70	
Point and Flex (*p*)	p. 179	
Zigzag Against a Wall (*p*)	p. 152	
Forward Bend (*y*)	p. 94	
Forward Bend Cobbler (*y*)	p. 99	
Mermaid (*p*)	p. 140	
Seated Spinal Twist (*y*)	p. 132	
Shoulder Stand (*y*) (if advanced)	p. 184	
Oblique Curl Up (*p*)	p. 89	
The Hundred (*p*)	p. 90	
Cat and Dog (*y*)	p. 198	
Resting Child (*p+y*)	p. 118	
Seated Relaxation (*y*)	p. 210	

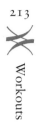

Four

Standing Posture (*y*)	p. 51	
Sun Salutation (*y*)	p. 200	
Waist Twist (*p*)	p. 128	
Triangle (*y*)	p. 148	
Cobbler (*y*)	p. 158	
Neck Rolls (*p*)	p. 70	
Curl Up (*p*)	p. 88	
Oblique Curl Up (*p*)	p. 89	
Rolling Down Cobra (*y*)	p. 204	
Dart (*p*)	p. 65	
Double Heel Kicks (*p*) or Single Heel Kicks (*p*)	p. 108 /106	
Downward Facing Dog (*y*)	p. 180	
Resting Child (*p+y*)	p. 118	
A Short Relaxation (*p*)	p. 208	

Five

Pelvic Stability – Knee Drops (*p*)	p. 62	
Starbugs (*p*)	p. 188	
Resting Child (*p+y*)	p. 118	
Bow and Arrow (*p*)	p. 126	
Forward Bend Cobbler (*y*)	p. 99	
Side Bend (*p*) or Mermaid (*p*)	p. 142 / 140	
King Pigeon (*y*)	p. 160	
Single Leg Stretch (*p*) Stage 1 or 2	p. 192	
Bridge (*y*)	p. 116	
Shoulder Stand (Advanced) (*y*)	p. 184	
Extended or Full Cobra (*y*)	p. 110 / 112	
Resting Child (*p+y*)	p. 118	
Seated Relaxation (*y*)	p. 210	

Six

Arm Openings (*p*)	p. 196	
Lying Down Spinal Twist (*y*)	p. 134	
Pelvic Stability – Knee Folds (*p*)	p. 62	
Ankle Circles (*p*)	p. 178	
Single Leg Stretch (*p*)	p. 192	
One-legged Seated Forward Bend (*y*)	p. 96	
Corkscrew (*p*)	p. 168	
Standing Side Bend (*y*)	p. 146	
Side-lying Quadriceps and Hip Flexor Stretch (*p*)	p. 154	
Diamond Press (*p*)	p. 102	
Extended Cobra (*y*)	p. 110	
Full Cobra (*y*) (if advanced)	p. 112	
Resting Child (*p+y*)	p. 118	

Seven

Starfish (*p*)	p. 184	
Lying Down Spinal Twist (*y*)	p. 134	
Neck Rolls (*p*)	p. 70	
The Hundred (*p*)	p. 90	
Locust (*y*)	p. 114	
Dumb Waiter (*p*)	p. 166	
Triangle (*y*)	p. 148	
Downward Facing Dog (*y*)	p. 180	
Crescent Moon (*y*)	p. 162	
Threading a Needle (*p*)	p. 170	
Cat and Dog (*y*)	p. 198	
Single Heel Kicks (*p*)	p. 106	
Resting Child (*p+y*)	p. 118	
Sun Salutation (*y*)	p. 200	
A Short Relaxation (*p*)	p. 208	

8 Further information

Equipment and Clothing

Agoy

Yoga bags, belts and rubber, non-slip mats. Available exclusively on the internet (www.agoy.co.uk) or via mail order on +44 (0)20 8933 8421.

Body Control Clothing

A capsule collection of comfortable, hi-performance sportswear in a selection of colours and sizes. Available to buy on the internet (www.bodycontrolclothing.com) or via mail order on +44 (0)1858 469 588.

Pilates Equipment

For a wide range of Pilates equipment, books, videos and accessories, visit the Body Control Pilates® website at www.bodycontrol.co.uk or call +44 (0)20 7379 3734.

Associations

Pilates

For details of your nearest qualified Body Control Pilates teacher, send a stamped addressed envelope to:

The Body Control Pilates® Association
PO Box 29061
London WC2H 9TB
England
Or visit the Body Control Pilates® website at www.bodycontrol.co.uk

Yoga

For details of your nearest qualified yoga teacher, contact the British Wheel of Yoga on +44 (0)1529 306 851.

Other Body Control Pilates Books

These are available from all good bookshops, or can be ordered from:

Book Services By Post
PO Box 29
Douglas,
Isle of Man IM99 1BQ.

Credit card hotline 01624 675 137
Postage and packing free in the UK.

Watch out for new titles!